CASE STUDIES IN

Emergency Nursing

EDITED BY

BARBARA MLYNCZAK-CALLAHAN, RN, MS, CCRN

Director of Nursing
Department of Emergency Medicine
The Johns Hopkins Hospital
Baltimore, Maryland

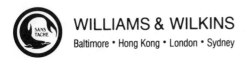
WILLIAMS & WILKINS
Baltimore • Hong Kong • London • Sydney

Editor: Susan M. Glover
Associate Editor: Marjorie Kidd Keating
Copy Editor: Lucy Mullins
Designer: Wilma E. Rosenberger
Illustration Planner: Ray Lowman
Production Coordinator: Anne Stewart Seitz

Printed in the United States of America

Library of Congress Cataloging-in-Publication Data

Case studies in emergency nursing / edited by Barbara Mlynczak-Callahan.
    p. cm.
    Includes bibliographical references.
    ISBN 0-683-01395-5
    1. Emergency nursing—Case studies.   2. Nursing assessment—Case studies.
    1. Mlynczak-Callahan, Barbara.
    [DNLM: 1. Emergencies—nursing—case studies.   2. Nursing Assessment.
    WY 154 C3368]
RT120.E4C37 1990
610.73'61—dc20
DNLM/DLC
for Library of Congress   89-21477
                                        CIP

                                 90 91 92 93 94
          1   2   3   4   5   6   7   8   9 10

PREFACE

This manual is not about how to make a medical or nursing diagnosis. However, it is about critical thinking and the diagnostic reasoning process that occurs from the moment the patient presents for help in the emergency department (ED) to his or her admission or discharge from the hospital. Organizing this reasoning process by health system acuity and nursing diagnoses assists the nurse in making life-or-death decisions about patient care even when the etiology is unclear. The authors of these case studies have been selected because of their expertise in emergency care and diagnostic reasoning. The case study format has been chosen because it lends itself to "thinking" through the major considerations for each patient type. Although protocols may vary from hospital to hospital or among prehospital care regions, rationale are provided for the specific interventions that are used in this manual based on an understanding of the etiology and pathophysiology of disease and the current standard of care for patients with similar complaints.

The cases included here are not intended to be all-inclusive of the myriad of patient complaints that are seen in the ED setting. The case studies here were selected to represent high-risk situations that may be encountered in any ED. These cases are fairly representative of situations encountered with high frequency in a selected urban setting. In other EDs across the country these conditions may be present but volume or frequency may not be the same.

However, the process of patient assessment and determination of acuity by presenting symptoms and the application of nursing diagnoses with an understanding of the etiology and pathophysiology of the presenting complaint can be applied to any patient situation and drive decision making for appropriate nursing intervention. Hopefully, this manual sets the stage for that process in any clinical setting. The reader is referred to other volumes in this series for case studies in trauma and critical care that are part of this framework of thinking.

I would be remiss if I did not take this opportunity to thank a few key people who helped make this production possible—Susan Glover for thinking of us; Diann for her tolerance of all my last minute changes; Shannon, who did not know she could type; and my husband Dan for his endless patience. A very special thank you is due to all those doctors, nurses, and pre-hospital providers who are out there daily, trying to make a difference.

Barbara Mlynczak-Callahan, RN, MS, CCRN

CONTRIBUTORS

Karla Alwood, MS, CRNP
Johns Hopkins University
School of Hygiene and Public Health
Department of Epidemiology
Baltimore, Maryland

Laurel Ann Ault, RN, BS
Child Abuse Liaison Nurse
Emergency Department
Union Memorial Hospital
Baltimore, Maryland

Kathleen J. Barnett, RN, MSN, CEN
Clinical Nurse Specialist
Department of Emergency Medicine
Johns Hopkins Hospital
Baltimore, Maryland

Valerie A. Barron, RN, BSN, CCRN, CEN
Staff Nurse
Chest Pain Emergency Department
St. Agnes Hospital
Critical Care Instructor
Homewood Hospital Center
Baltimore, Maryland

Patricia C. Bent, RN, CEN
Clinical Nurse
Department of Emergency Medicine
Johns Hopkins Hospital
Baltimore, Maryland

Carol A. Brown, MSW, LCSW
Senior Social Worker
Department of Emergency Medicine
Johns Hopkins Hospital
Baltimore, Maryland

Sharon A. Childs, RN, BSN, CEN
Graduate Student
Trauma/Critical Care Program
University of Maryland at Baltimore
Baltimore, Maryland

Patricia C. Epifanio, RN, MS, CEN
Emergency Nurse Coordinator
MIEMSS EMS Nursing and Specialty Care
Baltimore, Maryland

Suzanne P. Hangasky, RN, BS, CRNP
Nurse Practitioner
Department of Emergency Medicine
Johns Hopkins Hospital
Baltimore, Maryland

James Jay Hoelz, RN, MS, CEN
Head Nurse
Emergency Department
Mercer Medical Center
Trenton, New Jersey

Cynthia Kaczmarek, RN, BSN
Clinical Nurse
Department of Emergency Medicine
Johns Hopkins Hospital
Baltimore, Maryland

Kathleen Keenan, RN, MS, CCRN
Clinical Nurse Specialist
Department of Emergency Medicine
Johns Hopkins Hospital
Baltimore, Maryland

Debra Kosko, MN, CRNP
Clinical Coordinator
Maryland AIDS Professional Education
  Center
University of Maryland
Baltimore, Maryland

Laura Ann Kress, RN, BSN
Head Nurse
Department of Emergency Medicine
Johns Hopkins Hospital
Baltimore, Maryland

Debra Lanouette, RN, MSN, CS
Psychiatric Clinical Specialist
Department of Emergency Medicine
Johns Hopkins Hospital
Baltimore, Maryland

**Barbara Mlynczak-Callahan, RN, MS,
  CCRN**
Director of Nursing
Department of Emergency Medicine
Johns Hopkins Hospital
Baltimore, Maryland

Leticia V. M. Nanda, RN, MS
Senior Clinical Nurse
Wilmer Eye Institute
Johns Hopkins Hospital
Baltimore, Maryland

Ronald Nichols, RN
Registered Nurse/Assessment Specialist
Program for Alcohol and Other Drug
  Dependencies
Johns Hopkins Hospital
Baltimore, Maryland

Susan C. Roberson, RN, MSN, CRNP
Senior Nurse Practitioner
Department of Emergency Medicine
Johns Hopkins Hospital
Baltimore, Maryland

Cathy Robey-Williams, RN, MS, CCRN
Senior Clinical Nurse
Department of Emergency Medicine
Johns Hopkins Hospital
Instructor
Department of Emergency Health Services
University of Maryland Baltimore County
Baltimore, Maryland

Polly Thornton, RN
Staff Nurse
Emergency Department
St. Agnes Hospital
Baltimore, Maryland

Barbara Van de Castle, RN, MSN
Clinical Nurse
Department of Emergency Medicine
Johns Hopkins Hospital
Baltimore, Maryland

Kathleen A. Williams, RN, BSN
Clinical Research Nurse
Department of Cardiology
Johns Hopkins Hospital
Baltimore, Maryland

CONTENTS

Chapter
4 Gastrointestinal-Genitourinary (Elimination) and Nutrition Health Systems

Chapter
5 Structural Health System

INTRODUCTION

Barbara Mlynczak-Callahan, RN, MS, CCRN

Emergency nursing care is still in evolution, having first started in out of the way rooms in out of the way places in many hospitals. Only in recent years has the delivery of emergency care been recognized as a needed and valued component of the community and hospital's care delivery system. Rooms have been expanded and there is recognition of emergency departments (EDs). Medical and nursing organizations have developed to recognize the special education and training required for an individual to provide care in an emergency setting. Although many hospitals still staff their ED with "moonlighters" from other specialties, recognition of programs in emergency medicine are coming to the forefront. For nurses, the road has been bumpy as the nurse grapples with an identity that is not quite med-surg, not quite critical care. The Emergency Nurses Association has organized to validate the practice of emergency nursing through standards of practice and care. Emergency nursing practice is a unique opportunity to use and enhance the nursing process skills of anyone willing to be challenged. Emergency nursing practice also challenges the nurse to practice holistic nursing, under emotional conditions in very limited periods of time.

Case studies in this manual take into consideration two aspects of the emergency care structure that have a tremendous impact on practice: (1) the patient generally presents with a complaint of illness or signs and symptoms, rarely with a statement of medical diagnosis; (2) the patient is usually seen first by a nurse who must determine how acutely ill or potentially ill the patient is, and then what resources are appropriate to mobilize to manage that patient's care. Given these factors, a framework for nursing triage based on clustering of complaints, signs, and symptoms by health system and nursing care management based on related nursing diagnoses is used as an organizing model for patient assessment, intervention, and evaluation.

The framework used to organize the case studies for this manual is adapted from the model first introduced at The Johns Hopkins Hospital, Baltimore, Maryland, under the leadership of Reitz in 1982 (1). The model incorporates concepts of health and the dynamics of health status along with the nurse's role in assessing a patient's needs and intervening appropriately. The framework organizes health data into health dimensions and functional health systems. These health systems are further organized into biophysical health functions and behavioral health functions.

Using this framework for patient triage, clustering of symptoms by health systems, and then further organizing the assessment data by degrees of acuity provides a basis for prioritizing care for patients in the ED. This model for triage is adapted from that first organized by Christmyer, Catanzariti, Langford, and Reitz (2) and implemented in their ED. This health parameter concept for use in the ED is not unlike that described by Corrigan (3) which was adapted from the functional health parameter concept presented by Gordon for use with nursing diagnoses (4). The introduction of nursing diagnosis as a means of organizing nursing interventions and evaluating outcomes is a viable enhancement to the nursing process in the ED setting.

The nursing diagnoses chosen for presentation in this manual are based on those endorsed by the Seventh National Conference General Assembly of the North American Nursing Diagnosis Association (NANDA) in 1988.

In this manual, the overview for each chapter discusses the organization of patient complaints and symptoms into biophysical and psychosocial health systems based on this framework for holistic patient care. Levels of acuity are described as they relate to the severity of the patient's illness and consumption of nursing resources to provide care. A general description of the meaning of the acuity levels in the ED setting is presented in Table I. The overview of the health system is then followed by case studies that represent types of patients who are frequently seen in the emergency setting, triaged by health system complaint. Cases are designed to address the patient's chief complaint or symptoms, his or her acuity level, the etiology and physiology of symptoms, pertinent nursing diagnoses for the ED nurse to consider, and independent and interdependent nursing actions to be taken.

As is reasonable, a complete health assessment of the patient is conducted at triage that considers the biophysical, behavioral, and social health needs of the patient. The patient's acuity level is driven by the health system of highest acuity in the cluster of patient symptoms. For example, the patient with normal vital signs may be considered acuity level I in the circulatory health system. However, the patient's report of excruciating headache may rank as acuity level III in both the neurological-cerebral health system and sensory health system, identifying the patient as needing expeditious care.

Nursing diagnoses can be determined by analyzing the data collected within each health system and relating those data to the defining character-

Table 1 Leveling Process for Differentiating Nursing Acuity Related to Patient Health Systems

Level I	A rating of "1" (minor) indicates minimal or minor care requirements. The patient is generally capable of self-care and may require only minor treatments and few medications. The patient is generally ambulatory, and is able to care for him- or herself without assistance; activity is not restricted. The patient exhibits no behavioral deviations but may require minimal health teaching and emotional support. Such patients are frequently referred to other "nonurgent" clinics and community resources for assistance.
Level II	A rating of "2" (moderate) indicates partial dependence on nursing staff for assistance; periodic observation, treatments, and medication are required. The patient may require some activity restriction and some assistance with daily activities. The patient may manifest occasional behavioral deviation, i.e., slight confusion. The patient requires periodic health education and emotional support. This patient may be referred to some other "nonurgent" clinic. More often the patient is provided with an intermediary level of intervention by the triage nurse and then asked to wait while care is provided to patients in more urgent need of care.
Level III	A rating of "3" (major) indicates a major dependence on nursing staff for assistance. The patient requires considerable restriction of activity; may require total assistance in daily activities; may be incontinent; and requires frequent observation, treatments, and medications. The patient manifests marked emotional needs, and may require use of protective devices and exhibit severe deviation in behavior, i.e., marked confusion, hyperactivity. The patient may require considerable instruction. Patients in this category frequently have significant potential for poor outcome or serious complications if their needs are not addressed in a timely fashion. These patients are given high priority for treatment.
Level IV	A rating of "4" (intensive) indicates requirement for close and continuous observation and monitoring. The patient may require life-saving measures administered promptly and constantly; the patient may exhibit symptoms of extreme behavioral deviation; requires rigid activity restriction. The patient is unstable and may be unconscious. Patients in this category require immediate intervention. Resuscitative measures are frequently undertaken. Medical and nursing resource utilization is maximized to reverse immediate signs and symptoms of catastrophe.

istics as described by NANDA. Nursing interventions are selected based on an understanding of the etiology and of pathophysiology of the patient's complaint. The nurse in the emergency setting must set priorities as to which diagnoses are most life- or health-threatening to the patient and take immediate action. All nursing diagnoses may not be addressed during the episodic visit. Prioritization must be realistic. Intervention and desired patient outcomes must be achievable. The patient's psychosocial and discharge needs must be considered as pertinent to the treatment plan. Before discharge the nurse must determine that the patient has the intellectual, emotional, financial, and social resources to follow the plan of care adequately. The nurse's knowledge of community resources can assist in providing patient care at home rather than in the hospital. Case files for patients who repeatedly require the services of the ED should be available to all health team members so that the plan of care for the patient can be consistent and dynamic, as needed. The health system framework with related nursing diagnoses makes this possible.

REFERENCES

1. Reitz JA: Toward a comprehensive nursing intensity index. Part I, Development. *Nurs Manage* 16(8):21–30, 1985.
2. Christmeyer CS, Catanzariti PM, Langford AM, Reitz J: Bridging the gap: theory to practice. Part I, clinical applications. *Nurs Manage* 19(8):42–50, 1988.
3. Corrigan JO: Functional health pattern assessment in the emergency department. *J Emerg Nurs* 12(3):163–167, 1986.
4. Gordon M: Nursing diagnosis: process and application. New York: McGraw-Hill, 1982.

CHAPTER 1

Neurological-Cerebral and Cognitive Health Systems

Overview

The neurological-cerebral health system is concerned with the body's ability to receive and respond to stimuli. This health system includes the functions of the brain and the nerves and the structures that support these. The neurological-cerebral health system review includes assessment of level of consciousness as well as mental status. Mental status is usually assessed through characteristics of speech, nature of thought processes, general behavior and appearance, orientation, and memory. Patients with primary motor sensory deficits related to disruption of the peripheral nervous system are evaluated in this health system as well as in the sensory health system. In addition, patients with functional psychoses such as delirium or schizophrenia may be classified as having an alteration in neurological-cerebral health. The cognitive health system addresses the individual's ability to process and transmit information based on developmental, educational, and physiological capabilities.

CUE WORDS

Neurological-Cerebral Health System

CENTRAL NERVOUS SYSTEM	MENTAL STATUS	LEVEL OF CONSCIOUSNESS	PERIPHERAL NERVOUS SYSTEM
brain damage	behavior/appearance	eye opening	numbness/tingling/pain
hyperactivity	memory	eye movements	paresthesia
intracranial pressure	orientation	motor response	hyperesthesia
meningeal signs	speech	pupil response	
protective reflexes	thought experiences	sleep pattern	
seizure activity		verbal response	
		loss of consciousness	

Cognitive Health System

RECEPTION	PROCESSING	TRANSMISSION
language	comprehension	communication
readiness	education	feedback
receptiveness	knowledge	learning
resistance	learning disability	return demonstration
sensory impairment	thought process	retention
	understanding	
	developmental level	

RELATED NURSING DIAGNOSES ▬▬▬▬▬
Neurological-Cerebral Health System

sensory perceptual alteration (specify)
sleep pattern disturbance
altered thought processes
potential for injury
dysreflexia

Cognitive Health System

knowledge deficit
altered growth and development
decisional conflict
impaired verbal communication
altered thought processes
potential for injury

Department of Emergency Medicine Triage Protocols

Neurological-Cerebral Health System[a]

Level I	Level II	Level III	Level IV
Neck strain, no neurological deficits, no spinal tenderness	Hit head, no LOC; no vomiting; no neurological deficits; no spinal tenderness; able to ambulate	Hit head/neck, questionable LOC; alert; GCS 15 now; generalized weakness but able to move all extremities; PERRL; no spinal tenderness	Major trauma to head/neck; change in level of consciousness; unable to walk; vomiting; double/blurry vision; combative; spinal tenderness; unequal grips
	Known seizure disorder, out of medication, needs Rx; positive ETOH use, feels shaky, no tremors	Known seizure disorder; seizure prior to ED visit; not postictal; no seizure activity present; tremors	Active seizure state or postictal; experiencing aura; febrile, hallucinations, severe tremors
Minor headache with no associated symptoms		Headache, patient irritable, holds head; photophobia; appears uncomfortable; not relieved by OTC drugs; nausea and/or vomiting	Appears in acute distress, describes "worst headache I've ever had"; altered sensorium; positive nuchal rigidity; hypertensive; h/o head trauma within last 2–3 weeks
	c/o Numbness/tingling in extremity; no facial droop; mild headache; h/o hypertension; no change in mental status, speech, or ability to understand; h/o syncope	Sudden onset of decrease or inability to use one side of body; change in mental status; facial drooping; inability to speak; may be confused	

Cognitive Health System

Level I	Level II	Level III	Level IV
Patient with some degree of mental retardation; unable to comply with instructions; patient presents for nonurgent problem, accompanied by a responsible adult	Dizziness, not orthostatic	Minor motor dysfunction, ataxia, mild spasms; lethargy; dizziness with orthostasis	New onset paraplegia/quadriplegia; new onset paresis; h/o any neurological motor or demyelinating diseases, i.e., MS, MD, CP, ALS
Child/adolescent with minor complaint accompanied by a responsible adult		Adolescent not accompanied by adult regardless of complaint	Mentally retarded patient presents for medical or surgical treatment and is noisy and/or disruptive
Deaf or deaf mute without ability to communicate—needs interpreter			Child < 12 years not accompanied by responsible adult regardless of complaint
Speaks no English—needs interpreter			

a Abbreviations: LOC, loss of consciousness; GCS, Glascow coma score; PERRL, pupils equal and reactive to light; Rx, prescription; ETOH, ethyl alcohol; ED, emergency department; OTC, over-the-counter; h/o, history of; c/o, complains of; MS, multiple sclerosis; MD, muscular dystrophy; CP, cerebral palsy; ALS, amyotrophic lateral sclerosis.

4

1.1 MIGRAINE HEADACHES
Cynthia A. Kaczmarek, RN, BSN

Barbara is a 35-year-old black female who comes to the emergency department (ED) with a severe headache that has lasted over 4 days. At triage, Barbara appears to be in acute distress. Unable to find a comfortable position, she is holding her head in her hands while rocking back and forth. Barbara's vital signs on arrival are temperature 98.6° F, pulse 90, respirations 28, and blood pressure (BP) 214/129. Barbara describes paresthesia on the right side of her body with some tingling and weakness in the right hand. She has a right facial droop. Barbara also complains of having had nausea and vomiting for this same 4-day period.

Triage Assessment, Acuity Level IV: Appears in acute distress, describes "worst headache," BP diastolic >115, and neurological deficits.

Barbara is brought immediately to the treatment area where she describes visual changes with streaking, flashing lines that began with the onset of her headache. Barbara states that her menses just finished prior to the onset of this attack, a usual precursor for her headache. Barbara also shares that she has been feeling "depressed" since she separated from her husband 2 months ago. Barbara's past medical history includes diagnosed migraine headaches with almost monthly visits to the ED. Hypertension and depression are also chronic problems for her.

Barbara's current medications include hydrochlorothiazide (HCTZ), verapamil, nortriptyline, Reglan, Phenergan, and Demerol. She is allergic to Compazine (seizures), Stadol and Thorazine (syncope), Inderal (rash), codeine and Dilaudid (nausea). Barbara's physical assessment is normal except for the described neurological dysfunctions.

Barbara is placed in a room that is darkened and away from the main flow of activity. She is started on an intravenous solution of normal saline at 250 ml/hr. While in the ED, Barbara receives a total of 450 mg of meperidine with 150 mg of Vistaril, all given intramuscularly, before any relief of her headache and symptoms is obtained. When Barbara is released from the ED, no prescriptions are given to her and she is instructed to have a follow-up with her private neurologist.

QUESTIONS AND ANSWERS

1. **What are migraine headaches?**

Headaches are one of the most common ailments affecting people in the United States. Approximately 20% of the population experiences a type of headache that can be classified as a migraine. Most migraine conditions begin in adolescence and affect females twice as often as males (1, 2). Research suggests that there is a family history associated with migraines.

The exact cause of migraines is still unknown. It is believed that migraines are of vascular origin affecting both the intracranial and extracranial arteries (2). A study done by Graham and Wolff in the late 1930s suggests that an unidentified substance causes a cascade of events that may include platelet aggregation and release of various substances such as platelets, serotonin, and kinins (1, 3). A symptomatic vasoconstriction occurs in response to these substances and is usually focal. This vasoconstriction is followed by a reactive vasodilation in the extracranial arteries which results in the throbbing pain that is associated with the migraine headache (1).

There are two types of migraine headaches: classic and common. Classic migraines occur in approximately 10% of patients with migraines. In most cases there is a prodromal phase which begins about 30 min prior to the actual headache. In this prodromal phase there is usually some sensory dysfunctions such as visual deficits, scatomas, tingling, and paresthesia (2). The headache usually has a rapid onset with pain that is unilateral. The pain tends to concentrate in the frontal region and may radiate. Patients often describe the pain as throbbing and in synchrony with their pulse (3). Some accompanying symptoms include nausea and vomiting and an increase in BP. The headache can last anywhere from several hours to several days. As this description would suggest, Barbara experiences classic migraine headaches. The neurological findings with Barbara's headaches such as the facial droop and tingling in the extremities can be associated with her high BP and the many pontine hemorrhage scars that have been found on CAT scans of her brain.

The common migraine headache features many of the same symptoms of the classic migraine. However, the prodromal phase is not as severe. The common migraine headache can produce many of the accompanying symptoms such as nausea and vomiting lasting for several hours to several days (3).

2. How is the diagnosis of migraine headache achieved?

The diagnosis of migraine headache is based largely on the patient's history and presentation. The physical exam is usually unremarkable (4). Lab studies are usually not helpful. Sometimes, as in the case of Barbara, a CAT scan will reveal hemorrhages that have occurred as the result of high BP or excessive vasodilation of the arterioles.

Important facts for the nurse to include in the assessment of the patient include when the headache began; any predisposing factors that the patient can relate to the onset of the headache such as stress, menses, or family crisis; and the duration and the quality of the pain. It is clear from Barbara's history that many of these factors are present for her. The patient should also be asked if any measures taken have been effective in helping to reduce the pain. The nurse also needs to be aware of the patient's BP as a possible cause for the neurological changes that the patient is experiencing.

3. **What nursing diagnoses should be considered in this patient presentation?**

Many different factors need to be assessed when identifying nursing diagnoses for the migraine patient. The patient presents because there is significant pain. The patient's nutritional status and complications of nausea and vomiting that accompany migraines should be considered. Social, environmental, and psychological factors that may have an effect on the patient also should be assessed.

Diagnosis: Pain related to reaction vasodilation of extracranial arteries associated with migraine headache

Desired patient outcome: The patient will state that there has been a reduction in pain; the patient will exhibit behavioral cues that are consistent with the relief of pain such as no more rocking or head holding.

Diagnosis: Fluid volume deficit related to nausea and vomiting

Desired patient outcome: The patient will take 2000 ml of fluids intravenously or orally; the patient will not experience orthostatic vital sign changes; the patient's skin turgor will improve, mucous membranes will be moist.

Diagnosis: Altered cerebral perfusion related to high BP and migraine phenomena

Desired patient outcome: The patient will have a reduction in BP of less than 100 mg Hg diastolic; the patient will describe resolution of the numbness and tingling of right hand; facial droop will resolve.

Diagnosis: Ineffective individual coping related to personal vulnerability in a situational crisis

Desired patient outcome: The patient will be able to identify personal strengths that may promote effective coping; the patient will state a plan for either accepting or changing the situation; the patient will be able to identify and access community resources that are available when she feels unable to cope.

4. **What are the medical and nursing care measures for the patient with a migraine headache?**

The care provided to Barbara is useful in the management of any patient with a migraine headache. The patient needs to be placed in a darkened room that is away from the center of activity, and disturbed as little as possible. Decreasing the neurological and sensory stimulation to the patient helps in reducing the intensity of the pain associated with the migraine headache. Vital signs, especially BP, should be monitored. Barbara's BP is significantly high and she is having pronounced neurological changes. A stroke may occur because of the high pressure. A patient, like Barbara, should be assessed for deterioration of neurological signs that may include a decreased level of consciousness, alterations in speech patterns, pupillary changes, and other signs associated with cerebral vascular accidents. For the patient with a migraine headache a rapid reduction in BP may help to alleviate these symptoms. The patient should be given antiemetics such as Compazine or Phenergan to help relieve some of the accompanying symptoms of nausea and vomiting. Since Barbara is allergic to Compazine, she was given Phenergan. Fluids should also be provided, either intravenously or by mouth.

Pain medications should be administered as ordered. Narcotic analgesics are usually not recommended in the management of migraines. Because of the frequency of migraine attacks with some patients, the continual use of narcotics for pain management may cause the patient to become narcotic dependent or tolerant. However, if the attack is intractable, then narcotic analgesia may be required (5).

One of the most widely used drugs for the treatment of migraines is ergotamine. It is believed that this drug works by constricting the already dilated cranial arteries (5). For best results, this drug needs to be taken not more than 30 min after the prodromal phase begins (5, 6). Ergotamine had been tried for Barbara in the past but did not work for several reasons. A side effect of ergotamine therapy is an elevation of BP that could ultimately result in decreased arterial blood flow and tissue ischemia (6). Also, if the patient experiences a migraine headache more than twice a month, a different form of therapy is usually recommended. Since Barbara has chronic hypertension and often has frequent migraine attacks, it was decided that this would not be a beneficial treatment for her.

A prophylactic treatment plan needs to be initiated if the patient experiences migraines more than twice a month. This plan includes a visit and follow-up appointments with one doctor, preferably a neurologist. With this plan of treatment the patient works with the doctor on a one-to-one basis to try to establish a treatment plan of medications that works best for the individual patient and thereby decreases the number of ED visits and provides for consistency in care when an ED visit is needed.

Calcium channel blockers such as verapamil have in recent years been shown to be effective in the management of the migraine patient by increasing blood flow and oxygen supply to the tissues (6). Antidepressants such as the tricyclic antidepressants Elavil and Amitril have also been shown to be useful in long-term care (6). Antidepressants have sedative actions. They also increase the serotonin uptake from the synapses (6) which is believed to play a role in the cause of migraines. These drugs are still under investigation for use as treatment for migraines.

Barbara is well known to the ED staff. Her treatment plan for her depression usually involves talking with the ED psychiatrist and trying to identify resources within herself and her community that can help her cope more effectively. Barbara was referred back to her community psychiatry program for ongoing help in managing her most recent personal crisis following discharge from the ED.

REFERENCES

1. Diamond S. Migraine headache: Working for the best outcome. *Postgrad Med* 81:174, 1987.
2. Lewis SM, Collier IC: Medical-surgical nursing: assessment and management of clinical problems. New York: McGraw-Hill, 1418, 1983.
3. Sandler M: Monoamines and migraine: a path through the woods. In: Diamond S, Dalessio D, Graham J, et al., eds. Vasoactive substances relevant to migraine. Springfield, IL: Charles C Thomas, 3–18, 1975.
4. Gunderson CH: Management of the migraine. *Am Fam Phys* 33:138–139, 1986.
5. Edmeads JG: Migraine. *Can Med Assoc J* 138:107–109, 1988.
6. Govoni LE, Hayes JE: Drugs and nursing implications. 5th ed. Norwalk, CT: Appleton-Century-Crofts, 66–67, 509, 1269, 1985.
7. Kim M, McFarland G, McLane A: Pocket guide to nursing diagnoses. St. Louis, C. V. Mosby, 1984.

1.2 SEIZURES: WHEN ALCOHOL IS THE CULPRIT

Kathleen J. Barnett, RN, MSN, CEN

Mr. H. is a 44-year-old white male who arrives in the ED after experiencing a generalized tonoclonic seizure at home, witnessed by his fiancée. The seizure occurred approximately 1 hr prior to arrival. Mr. H admits to a long history of alcohol (ethanol) abuse and has experienced previous withdrawal seizures, although he denies any history of delirium tremens or blackouts. He was previously on phenytoin, but has not been on it "for a long time." Mr. H. states he drank 4 quarts of beer the previous evening. He is anxious and tremulous, and ambulates with a cane. Vital signs at triage are BP 170/100, pulse 112, respirations 28, and temperature 37.6° C (99.6° F). Mr. H. is oriented to person, place, and time, but does not recall the President of the United States or other significant current events. Strength, sensation, and cranial nerves are intact, and reflexes are normal. However, Mr. H. has severe gait ataxia and minimal end-gaze nystagmus. Finger-to-nose coordination is slightly dysmetric. Sclera are injected, and there are significant dental caries. The neck is supple and lungs are clear; heart sounds reveal an S4 gallop. The abdomen is soft and nontender, with no masses or organomegaly. Mr. H. denies any illicit drug use, but smokes two packs of cigarettes a day.

Triage Assessment, Acuity Level III: Recent seizure activity and recent ethanol ingestion with history of alcohol withdrawal seizures; tremors; ataxia.

When Mr. H. is brought to the treatment area, a 1000 ml solution of 5% dextrose and 0.45% normal saline is started at 125 ml/hr with additives of 100 mg thiamine, 0.2 mg folic acid, and 2 g magnesium sulfate. Labwork is drawn simultaneously for a complete blood count (CBC), differential, electrolytes, calcium, magnesium, amylase, bilirubin, prothrombin time (PT), partial thromboplastin time (PTT), and ethanol level. Mr. H. is placed on a stretcher with side rails up in a well-lighted, high-observation area of the ED. A vest restraint is applied.

QUESTIONS AND ANSWERS

1. **What nursing diagnoses are applicable to this patient?**

    The patient with chronic alcohol abuse, alcohol withdrawal, or alcohol intoxication has a multitude of problems due to the multisystemic effects of the drug, including psychosocial complications. Obviously, not all nursing diagnoses can be addressed in the ED visit; however, the following diagnoses would likely be high on the priority list for the patient experiencing alcohol intoxication or withdrawal manifested by seizure activity.

    Diagnosis: Potential for injury related to seizures or to altered sensorium secondary to alcohol intoxication
    <u>Desired patient outcome:</u>   The patient will be seizure-free. If seizures recur, patient is in a safe environment that will protect him from falls or other injury.

    Diagnosis: Fluid volume deficit related to ethanol-induced diuresis and/or decreased fluid intake
    <u>Desired patient outcome:</u>   The patient maintains a heart rate less than 100 beats/min and systolic BP greater than 90 mm Hg. Urine output remains at greater than 30 ml/hr. Mucous membranes are moist.

    Diagnosis: Altered nutrition, less than body requirements, related to diminished dietary intake, diminished absorption of nutrients, and/or nonnutrient caloric intake
    <u>Desired patient outcome:</u>   Patient demonstrates improved nutritional status as indicated by appropriate lab values, particularly glucose, ketones, and magnesium.

    Diagnosis: Alteration in sensory-perceptual pattern related to central nervous system (CNS) depressant effects of ethanol or to hallucinations
    <u>Desired patient outcome:</u>   The patient will remain free of hallucinations or experience a reduction or cessation of hallucinations, if occurring. The patient will be alert and oriented.

    Diagnosis: Knowledge deficit of effects of alcohol on the body
    <u>Desired patient outcome:</u>   Patient is able to describe the relationship between alcohol and his symptoms, verbalize ways in

which some deleterious effects might be avoided, and state where he can be referred for detoxification.

2. **What is the basis for Mr. H.'s seizure and other neurological symptoms?**

A seizure is the sudden, recurrent transient disturbance in mental status, body movement, or both caused by excessive electrical discharges of brain cells. A seizure disorder is a symptom, not a disease. Mr. H.'s symptomatology is related to the adverse effects of chronic ethanol abuse, recent excesses, and acute withdrawal. Alcoholism is defined as the continuing of drinking despite physical, social, or occupational problems related to alcohol use.

After ethanol is ingested, it is primarily absorbed in the lumen of the small intestine, although a small amount is absorbed through the gastric mucosa. Numerous factors influence the rate of ethanol absorption, including the concentration of ethanol in the beverage, pH and buffering capacities of the beverage, concentrations of congeners (chemical components that affect color, taste, and aroma) in the beverage, gastric emptying time following ingestion, emotional state of the drinker, and type and amount of food ingested with or before ethanol (1, 2). Because ethanol is distributed throughout the body to all tissues based on their water content, persons with greater body mass or greater body water can ingest proportionately higher amounts of ethanol and still maintain lower intravascular and body tissue concentrations (1).

More than 90% of ethanol ingested is metabolized in the liver. Only 2 to 10% is excreted by the lungs or kidneys, although the amount of ethanol in expired air or urine is directly proportional to the blood alcohol concentration (BAC) (1). The ability of the liver to metabolize ethanol may increase significantly with increasing amount and duration of ethanol ingestion, as the enzymes in the liver for alcohol and drug metabolism increase. Because of this phenomenon, other drugs may show accelerated clearance in the alcoholic as well, including anticoagulants, anticonvulsants, antibiotics, and oral antidiabetic agents.

The alcohol withdrawal syndrome that occurs with patients who are alcoholics has been grouped into four stages of increasing severity (3). Although the patient in withdrawal does not necessarily go through all four stages, each stage has a distinct set of signs and symptoms that defines it.

Stage one occurs at 6 to 8 hr following cessation of alcohol intake. It is characterized by mild tremulousness, anxiety, nausea, vomiting, and insomnia. The patient may be diaphoretic and easily startled. Tachycardia, mild hypertension, and hyperreflexia may also be present.

In stage two, which usually begins at 24 hr after cessation or reduction of alcohol intake, the autonomic hyperactivity of stage one continues, but the patient experiences hallucinations. These are primarily auditory, but may also be visual, tactile, or olfactory.

Stage three of alcohol withdrawal generally occurs at 7 to 48 hr after reduction or cessation, and is characterized by seizures. One or more seizures may occur over several hours; more than half of patients who develop withdrawal seizures experience multiple seizures (4). If untreated, the seizures may progress to delirium tremens.

The onset of delirium tremens is the hallmark of stage four. Frequently seen 3 to 5 days after cessation or reduction of alcohol intake, delirium tremens are characterized by autonomic hyperactivity—tremors, diaphoresis, fever, hypertension, and tachycardia—and by illusions, hallucinations, and global confusion (3, 5).

3. **How can it be determined that Mr. H.'s seizure is ethanol-related? Isn't it possible that idiopathic epilepsy, head trauma, or other drug toxicities could be the cause of the seizures?**

It is certainly possible that Mr. H.'s seizure could be due to any one of a number of etiologic factors or to a combination of factors. For instance, it is possible that Mr. H.'s drinking has suppressed an epileptic cause for his seizure that becomes apparent when drinking stops. Alcohol withdrawal seizures are a diagnosis of exclusion. Any first-time seizure should appropriately receive hospital admission and a diagnostic workup. However, a number of factors will assist in determining if a seizure fits the pattern of alcohol withdrawal.

History of seizures and use of antiepileptic medications are indications of previous problems. The medical record should be referenced to confirm this, particularly if the patient is postictal or a poor historian. Mr. H. stated that he had taken phenytoin at an earlier time. Phenytoin may be given to a patient with ethanol withdrawal seizures, but only for a limited period as prophylaxis. The usefulness of phenytoin as a long-term maintenance therapy for the patient with alcohol withdrawal seizures has not been demonstrated (6). The major antiepileptic drugs are described in Table 1.2.1.

Alcohol withdrawal seizures are usually grand mal seizures, but of shorter duration than idiopathic seizures (7). Tongue biting and loss of sphincter control are less common in alcohol withdrawal seizures than in idiopathic seizures (8). The electroencephalogram (EEG) of the patient experiencing an alcohol withdrawal seizure will return to normal after seizure activity, whereas the EEG of a patient experiencing an idiopathic seizure will display abnormalities during and following the seizure (8). Focal seizures are not associated with alcohol withdrawal and necessitate workup to rule out a space-occupying

Table 1.2.1 Major antiepileptic drugs

Drug	Usual Maintenance Dose	Indications	Side Effects	Toxic Signs
phenytoin (Dilantin)	4–8 mg/kg/day i.v./p.o. in children; 300–400 mg/day i.v.-/p.o. in adults	tonicoclonic/complex partial/status epilepticus	gingival hyperplasia, rash, hirsutism, facial coarsening, fever, exfoliative dermatitis, leukopenia	nystagmus, ataxia, drowsiness, tremors, nausea, constipation
phenobarbital	5–10 mg/kg/day i.v./i.m./p.o. in children; 90–180 mg/day i.v./i.m./p.o. in adults	tonoclonic/complex partial/elementary partial	rash, physical dependence	sedation, psychic changes, nystagmus, ataxia
primidone (Mysoline) Largely converted to phenobarbital in blood, especially when used as adjunctive therapy	10–20 mg/kg/day p.o. in children; 750–1500 mg/day p.o. in adults	tonoclonic/complex partial/elementary partial	rash, physical dependence	sedation, psychic changes, nystagmus, ataxia, gastrointestinal disturbance
carbamazepine (Tegretol)	400–1000 mg in children; 400–1200 mg in adults	complex partial/tonoclonic/elementary partial	lethargy (less common), depressed erythropoiesis, lens opacities	diplopia, dizziness, nausea/vomiting, ataxia

13

lesion resulting from head trauma or other pathology (9). A close examination of the head and neck should be performed to detect any external signs of trauma in a patient with seizures.

4. **What nursing interventions would be appropriate to initiate in this situation?**

Mr. H. presents with a history of alcohol withdrawal seizures, recent ingestion of alcohol, and a witnessed seizure prior to arrival. This combination of factors makes it apparent that Mr. H. continues to be at risk for further seizure activity. Mr. H. should be placed in a well-lighted, high-observation area of the ED. Precautions should be taken to prevent injury to Mr. H. should another seizure occur—side rails should be up, padded, and stretcher wheels should be locked. Mr. H. should be placed on his side to allow drainage of secretions in the event of seizure, and airway equipment should be readily available. A vest restraint may be indicated for some patients, as seizure activity can be violent and bring a patient off a stretcher.

The presence of tremors, ataxia, and anxiety, and the automatic hyperactivity demonstrated by hypertension and tachycardia all point to the need for sedation for Mr. H. Recognition of the signs and symptoms of alcohol withdrawal and prompt sedation of the patient will prevent worsening of symptoms and hopefully prevent further seizure activity. The benzodiazepines are generally recognized as the drug of choice for alcohol withdrawal symptoms, with chlordiazepoxide and diazepam the most commonly used agents. Intramuscular absorption of these two drugs is erratic and unreliable; therefore this route should be avoided. Oxazepam is available for oral administration and has a shorter half-life than either chlordiazepoxide or diazepam. Reassurance is also an important component in allaying the anxiety and fear that are associated with alcohol withdrawal.

Vital-sign monitoring will be essential for Mr. H. All his vital-sign parameters are outside normal limits on his admission to the ED. Frequent monitoring will assist in determining if Mr. H. is returning to a normal baseline or if he is progressing further in the alcohol withdrawal syndrome.

Initiation of intravenous hydration and supplementation of intravenous fluid with vitamins and magnesium are necessary. The chronic alcoholic not only faces the volume depletion caused by diuresis and inadequate fluid intake, but also malnutrition from diminished intake and absorption of protein, B vitamins (especially folic acid and thiamine), and certain minerals. Alcohol also increases urinary losses of amino acids, magnesium, potassium, and zinc. Administration of intravenous fluid with magnesium, thiamine, and folate or multivitamin additives should be standard therapy for the chronic alcoholic with withdrawal symptoms. Glucose should be given to *any* unconscious patient in the ED to rule out hypoglycemia; in the malnourished chronic alcoholic glucose provides carbohydrate calories as well.

TIP: Thiamine is a coenzyme in the metabolism of glucose, and should always be given prior to glucose in the chronic alcoholic patient to prevent precipitation of Wernicke-Korsakoff syndrome, which is manifested by oculomotor abnormalities, nystagmus, ataxia of gait, and global confusion. Thiamine can be safely given intravenously either directly or by infusion in most intravenous solutions.

TIP: A finger stick (Dextrostix) blood glucose should be checked routinely on all patients who present with seizure. Seizures can cause hypoglycemia; hypoglycemia can cause seizures.

TIP: Chronic alcohol consumption causes total body depletion of magnesium stores, which in turn decreases the seizure threshold. The serum magnesium level may not accurately reflect the degree of depletion; a standard dose of 1 g magnesium is generally acceptable for a chronic alcoholic patient.

Neurological monitoring is also essential for the patient in alcohol withdrawal. Serial neurological checks will provide information on Mr. H.'s progress or deterioration with regard to the desired patient outcomes. The patient's orientation, general level of consciousness, degree and location of tremors, presence or absence of hallucinations, speech, and thought processes are all significant parameters to assess. Reorientation of the patient at frequent intervals should also be part of the nurse's interventions.

Before being discharged from the ED, Mr. H. should have achieved the desired outcomes as identified in the nursing plan of care. He and his family should be encouraged to seek assistance through follow-up care and to establish a regular care provider to restore his normal body functions. A detoxification referral is made, although Mr. H. has not given clear indications that he is ready for such a program.

REFERENCES

1. Mendelson JH In: Biochemical pharmacology of alcohol. Efron DH, et al., eds. Psychopharmacology: a review of progress 1957–1967. PHS Publication #1836, U.S. Government Printing Office, Washington, D.C., 1968.

2. Iber FL: In alcoholism, the liver sets the pace. *Nutr Today* 6:1:2–9, 1971.

3. Behnke RH: Recognition and management of alcohol withdrawal syndrome. *Hosp Prac* 11:79–84, 1976.

4. Victor M, Adams RD: The effect of alcohol on the nervous system. *Research Publications—Association for Research in Nervous and Mental Disease* 32:526–623, 1953.

5. Brown CG: The alcohol withdrawal syndrome. *Ann Emerg Med* 11:276–280, 1982.

6. Josephson GW, Sabatier HS: Rational management of alcohol withdrawal seizures. *South Med J* 71:1095–1097, 1978.

7. Victor M: A study of epilepsy in the alcoholic patient. In: Simmeon L, ed. Modern neurology. Boston: Little, Brown, and Co., 555–576, 1979.

8. Talbott GD, Gander O: Convulsive seizures in the alcoholic: a clinical appraisal from the Baltimore Public Inebriate Program. *Md St Med J* 23:81–85, 1974.

9. Victor M: Treatment of alcoholic intoxication and the withdrawal syndrome. *Psychosom Med* 28:636–650, 1966.

1.3 ALTERED MENTAL STATUS: TRICYCLIC ANTIDEPRESSANT DRUG OVERDOSE

Barbara Mlynczak-Callahan, RN, MS, CCRN

Rachel is a 26-year-old black female who is brought into the ED and is unresponsive to painful stimuli. The paramedics radioed ahead that the patient was found by her mother unconscious in her room. The patient's mother found an empty bottle of amitriptyline at Rachel's side. The amitriptyline was the mother's prescription that the mother had filled at the pharmacy the previous day, a supply of thirty 100-mg pills. On arrival to the ED the patient's BP is 90/40, pulse 144, respirations 6 and shallow. Her skin is warm and dry; her muscle tone is myoclonic. She is immediately taken to the resuscitation area for airway management, fluid resuscitation, and poisoning detoxification.

Triage Assessment, Acuity Level IV: Loss of consciousness, systolic BP < 90 mm Hg, pulse > 120 beats/min; respiratory rate < 12.

QUESTIONS AND ANSWERS

1. **What is the immediate response of the ED nursing staff in the management of the patient with a drug overdose with loss of consciousness and significant cardiovascular instability?**

Rapid evaluations of the patient's airway, breathing, and circulation are the essential first activities in the management of the poisoned patient. For a patient such as Rachel who has a significant reduction in level of consciousness, protecting the patient's airway is critical. It is not unusual to move quickly to assist the physician to manually intubate and mechanically ventilate the patient.

The patient's BP and heart rate are monitored closely for abnormalities, and volume expanders are given for significant hypotension. In virtually all cases of coma or altered mental status, the nurse should also anticipate the physician to order the following agents: glucose, 25 g to be administered intravenously over 3 to 4 min; naloxone (Narcan), 0.8 to 2 mg or 0.005 to 0.03 mg/kg intravenous push, repeated as many as 2 to 5 times (1). If alcoholism or malnutrition is suspected, 100 mg thiamine may be administered intravenously or intramuscularly. If the patient is experiencing seizures, intravenous diazepam or phenytoin may be indicated. Correction of acidosis, hypoxemia, electrolyte abnormalities, hypoglycemia, and hypo- or hyperthermia is essential to the survival of the patient (2, 3). In the case of tricyclic antidepressant (TCA) overdose, some consideration has been given to the use of physostigmine to counteract the anticholinergic effects of the drug. However, onset of seizure activity is a frequent occurrence when physostigmine is used, and, therefore, this treatment modality should be used with caution (4, 5).

When the poison is unknown, additional assessments may be performed to determine the type of poisoning that has occurred. The assessment includes changes in vital signs, ocular signs, breath odors, skin signs, cardiopulmonary signs, and altered muscle tone (Table 1.3.1) (1, 2, 3). A 12-lead ECG should be obtained to assist with further differential diagnosis (Table 1.3.2) (1, 2, 3). Routine blood samples obtained should include cell counts, electrolytes, glucose, ketones, liver and renal function indices, prothrombin time, arterial blood gases, and blood urine samples for toxicology screens. If the poison was ingested by mouth, a stomach wash is indicated for lab analysis of stomach contents. A chest x-ray is indicated to evaluate for pulmonary edema that could be caused by narcotics, barbiturates, salicylates, ethchlorvynol, or corrosive chemicals (1, 2). Infiltrates may be present caused by aspiration of gastric contents or inhalation of metal fumes or hydrocarbons.

Table 1.3.1 Physical findings associated with various types of poisons

Altered vital signs
  Hypertension: amphetamines, phencyclidine, phenylpropanolamine, anticholinergics, cocaine, nicotine
  Hypotension: sedative-hypnotics, narcotics, antihypertensives, theophylline, clonidine, β-blockers, tricyclic antidepressants, nonspecific autonomic nervous dysfunction with venous pooling
  Hyperthermia: salicylates, amphetamines, phencyclidine, anticholinergics, seizures due to any cause, toxic psychosis
  Hypothermia: narcotics, barbiturates, ethanol, other sedative-hypnotics, clonidine, phenothiazines
  Hyperpnea: salicylates or other agents causing metabolic acidosis
  Tachycardia: amphetamines, cocaine, caffeine, atropine, tricyclic antidepressants
  Bradycardia: pilocarpine, *Amanita muscaria* mushrooms, organophosphates, β-blockers, antidysrhythmics
Ocular signs
  Miosis (pinpoint pupils): narcotics, clonidine, organophosphates, phenothiazines, deep sedative-hypnotic overdose, pilocarpine, pontine or cerebellar hemorrhage
  Mydriasis (dilated pupils): anticholinergics, amphetamines, cocaine, LSD, glutethimide, ophthalmic drops
  Nystagmus: phenytoin, phencyclidine (especially vertical nystagmus), alcohol, many sedative-hypnotics
  Ophthalmoplegia: botulism, sedative-hypnotics

Oculogyric crisis: haloperidol, other antipsychotics
Optic neuritis: methanol
Breath odors
   Smoke: fire-associated toxins
   Garlic: arsenic, arsine gas, organophosphates
   Bitter almond or silver polish: cyanide
   Wintergreen: methyl salicylate
   Pearlike: chloral hydrate
   Rotten eggs: hydrogen sulfide
   Acetone: diabetic ketoacidosis, isopropanol
   Typical odors of ethanol, ammonia, tobacco, disinfectants, camphor, glue, paraldehyde
Skin signs
   Phlebitis, needle tracks: parental drug abuse
   Cyanosis: ergotamine, agents causing hypoxemia, hypotension, or methemoglobinemia
   Flushed, red: carbon monoxide (rare), cyanide (rare), anticholinergics, boric acid
   Acneiform rash: bromides, chlorinated aromatic hydrocarbons
   Bullae: nonspecific for sedative-hypnotic overdose, carbon monoxide, and other causes of
     coma
   Diaphoresis: hypoglycemia, organophosphates, salicylates
Cardiopulmonary signs
   Rhythm disturbance: tricyclic antidepressants, phenothiazines, analeptics
   Rhonchi/wheezing: inhalational agents, aspiration of hydrocarbons (or vapors) or caustic
     agents, aspiration of gastric contents
   Wheezing/pulmonary edema: narcotics, anticholinergics, muscarinic agonists, cholinesterase
     inhibitors
Altered muscle tone
   Increased: amphetamines, phencyclidine, antipsychotics
   Flaccid: sedative-hypnotics, narcotics, clonidine
   Fasciculations: organophosphates, lithium
   Rigidity: haloperidol, phencyclidine, strychnine
   Dystonic posturing: antipsychotics, phencyclidine
   Tremor: lithium, nicotine, or stimulant overdose; alcohol or sedative-hypnotic withdrawal
   Asterixis (flapping tremor): agents causing hepatic encephalopathy
   Seizures: tricyclic antidepressants, theophylline, amphetamines, cocaine, phencyclidine,
     phenothiazines, isoniazid, lindane, other chlorinated hydrocarbons and pesticides

Table 1.3.2 Electrocardiographic manifestations of poisoning

Sign	Possible Cause (Drugs, Toxins, or Underlying Condition)
Prolonged QT interval	Arsenic
	Hypocalcemia (ethylene glycol)
	Phenothiazines
	Tricyclic antidepressants
	Type I antidysrhythmic agents
Prolonged QRS interval	Phenothiazines (selected)
	Tricyclic antidepressants
	Type I antidysrhythmic agents
Atrioventricular block	Beta-adrenergic blockers
	Calcium channel-blocking agents
	Digitalis glycosides
	Tricyclic antidepressants
	Type I antidysrhythmic agents

Ventricular tachydysrhythmias

Amphetamines
Cocaine
Digitalis glycosides
Theophylline
Tricyclic antidepressants
Type I antidysrhythmic agents

Ischemic pattern or current of injury

Cellular asphyxiants (cyanide, monoxide)
Hypoxemia (pneumonia)
Hypotension

---

2. **What are the various methods used to eliminate poisons from the gastrointestinal (GI) tract?**

The overall outcome or prognosis of the orally poisoned patient is often related to the rapid removal of the poison from the GI tract. The nurse can expect to begin the process of elimination of ingested toxins for the patient as soon as the patient's vital functions have stabilized. Elimination methods are designed to empty the stomach both anterograde and retrograde before significant intestinal absorption of the toxin can occur. Stomach emptying can occur by induced emesis or lavage. However, studies have shown that there is only 30% retrieval of stomach contents using this method (6). Intestinal absorption and movement of some substances can be decreased by the use of neutralizers, activated charcoal, and cathartics.

There are major contraindications to the induction of emesis in patients such as Rachel with a significant reduction in level of consciousness. Aspiration is quite likely to occur. Other contraindications to induced emesis are after ingestion of caustic agents, ingestion of hydrocarbons, presence of seizures, loss of gag reflex, and known patient sensitivity to agents such as ipecac and apomorphine (7). Further, if activated charcoal and cathartics are to be used to decrease toxin absorption, the drugs used to induce emesis may lead the patient to vomit the charcoal reducing its effectiveness.

Gastric lavage is a useful technique for emptying the stomach. The nurse can anticipate the need to pass a large lavage tube, usually 32 French (FR) in diameter. The nurse should assess that the patient's airway is protected during this process and that the appropriate placement of the tube has been confirmed by the physician on x-ray. Lavage is performed by serially instilling water or normal saline and then withdrawing the fluid along with the other gastric contents. Normal saline is universally recognized as safe, while tap H_2O may provide a convenient and inexpensive alternative (8). Studies (9) suggest that adult patients can tolerate water lavage without depleting serum electrolytes. This lavage should continue until the fluid returns clear.

Once the lavage is complete, the tube may be used for the administration of charcoal, cathartics, or neutralizers.

TIP: Use of activated charcoal is the most frequent and effective method for poison control in the ED patient.

Activated charcoal acts by absorption of the toxin through pores in the charcoal particles and subsequent chemical binding to the pore walls. Activated charcoal does not bind well to elemental metals such as lead, lithium, boron, and iron; boric acid; cyanide; strong acids or alkalis; ethanol; petroleum distillates; or certain pesticides (6). Other therapeutic actions must be taken under these conditions. The optimal ratio of activated charcoal to ingested drug is 10 to 1. When the amount of drug ingested is unknown, the recommended dosages are 20 to 25 g for children and 50 to 100 g for adults (6, 7, 10). The newer preparations of activated charcoal are combined with a cathartic, hurrying the compound through the intestine, thereby minimizing absorption of the toxin. Contraindications for use of activated charcoal and cathartics are intestinal obstruction and ileus. Since Rachel ingested an anticholinergic agent that decreases peristalsis, ongoing assessment of her abdomen, including distention and bowel sounds, is critical.

Other methods to clear drugs that have already been absorbed in the blood stream are forced diuresis and control of urine pH, and in more extreme cases hemodialysis or hemoperfusion. For some chemicals there are specific antidotes and your regional "poison control center" can be very helpful in management and treatment of the poisoned patient.

3. **Since we have a strong indication that Rachel has taken an overdose of a TCA medication, what should be our special considerations in her care and management?**

TCAs are closely related to phenothiazines which share degrees of anticholinergic, adrenergic, and α-blocking properties (3, 10). Anticholinergic effects include mydriasis, dry mucous membranes, tachycardia, urinary retention, and decreased peristalsis. Thermoregulation is affected and the patient may be either hypo- or hyperthermic. If the patient is awake, she is usually confused and agitated and may have hallucinations. Frequently, like Rachel, these patients report to the ED comatose with hyperreflexia, myoclonic movements, and, occasionally, grand mal seizures. Cardiotoxicity is a frequent and significant occurrence and includes tachycardia, disturbances of intraventricular conduction, ventricular arrhythmias, atrioventricular conduction defects, profound bradycardia, and cardiac arrest (11, 12). Myocardial contractility is also effected and can cause significant hypotension. Phenytoin (Dilantin) appears to be the drug of choice for managing patients with cardiovascular complications in TCA overdose. In doses of 5 to 7 mg/kg body weight, phenytoin enhances atrioventricular and intraventricular conduction as well as decreases ventricular automaticity (3, 13, 14, 15). Continuous cardiac monitoring by the nurse is essential in identifying early changes in QRS morphology or duration. Ongoing evaluation of BP and HR is also indicated.

An interesting variable in the care of the patient with a TCA overdose is that there can be a delay in symptom occurrence or symptoms can recur after early improvement (3). Arrhythmias and conduction blocks have been reported to recur after several hours of patient stability and up to 12 days later. Therefore, the emergency nurse must be continuously vigilant for these changes (11, 12).

4. **What are the essential nursing diagnoses to be considered in the care of Rachel?**

    Since Rachel has presented comatose with significant alteration in her cardiac function, she is at immediate risk for cardiopulmonary arrest and complications of hypoxia and aspiration. Critical nursing diagnoses include:

    Diagnosis: Ineffective airway clearance related to reduced alertness and suppression of gag reflex from CNS-depressant effects of the medication

    Desired patient outcome: The patient will maintain a patent airway; the patient will have a respiratory rate of 12 to 24, and clear breath sounds; the patient will expectorate secretions effectively.

    Diagnosis: Impaired gas exchange related to slow shallow respirations from CNS-depressant effects of the medication

    Desired patient outcome: The patient will have ventilation and gas exchange maintained. The patient will have clear breath sounds, respiratory rate of 12 to 24, and pink mucous membranes.

    Diagnosis: Altered cerebral and cardiopulmonary tissue perfusion, related to decreased arterial blood flow from depressant effects on the myocardium of the overdosed medication

    Desired patient outcome: The patient will achieve improved mental alertness and orientation to person, place, and time; skin will be warm and dry; urinary output > 30 ml/hr; systolic BP ≥ 90 mm Hg; HR ≤ 100 beats/min.

    Diagnosis: Hopelessness manifested by suicidal action, etiology unknown

Desired patient outcome: The patient will discuss reasons for the overdose and identify precipitating factors. The patient will describe strategies and resources available to manage stress and enhance coping. The patient will display coping behaviors that are health promoting such as participating in self-care and care planning.

Diagnosis: Violence, self-directed, etiology unknown

Desired patient outcome: The patient will not direct further violence at self. The patient will describe strategies to manage feelings of violence toward self and will identify available resources to assist with management of violent feelings.

Diagnosis: Ineffective family coping related to inadequate understanding of situation; feelings of guilt, grief, fear

Desired patient outcome: The patient's mother will ask appropriate questions and state a realistic understanding of current crisis situation. The patient's mother will state that feelings of guilt, grief, and fear are normal. The patient's mother will identify other family members and/or friends who can be of support.

5. **What further care is indicated for Rachel based on these diagnoses?**

Rachel will probably be admitted to a critical care unit for ongoing assessment and management. The ED nurse should ensure that her vital signs are continuously monitored, that her airway is protected, and that her oxygenation remains stable. Her family is in need of emotional support, and arrangements should be made for them to receive counseling and assistance either from a social worker, psychiatric counselor, or clergy. Rachel along with her family will need ongoing psychiatric support should she survive this event. The incidence of death in patients presenting with this degree of catastrophic deterioration from TCA overdose is high. The family should be provided with the appropriate emotional supports to help them to begin the process of grieving. The ED nursing report to the inpatient unit should include these arrangements.

REFERENCES

1. Bourg P, Sherer C, and Rosen P: Standardized nursing care plans for emergency departments. St. Louis: C.V. Mosby, 140, 1986.
2. Done AK: Poisoning—A systematic approach for the emergency department physician. Presented Aug. 6 to 9, 1979, at Snowmass Village, Colorado. Symposium sponsored by Rocky Mountain Poison Center.
3. Callaham M: Tricyclic antidepressant overdose. *JACEP* 8(10):413, 1979.

4. Pall H, Czeck K, Katzaurek R, et al.: Experiences with physostigmine salicylate in tricyclic antidepressant poisoning. *Acta Pharmacol Toxicol* 41:171–178, 1977.
5. Preskorn S, Irwin H: Toxicity of tricyclic antidepressants—kinetics, mechanism, intervention, a review. *J Clin Psychiatry* 43:151–156, 1982.
6. Dammann K: Activated charcoal. In: Tox talks. Charlottesville, Va.: Blue Ridge Poison Center 1(5):1–4, 1988.

7. Tintinalli JE, Rothstein FJ, Krome RL: Emergency medicine: a comprehensive study guide. New York: McGraw-Hill 285, 1985.

8. Johnston JB, ed: Tricyclic antidepressant overdose. In: Emergency nursing reports. Rockville, Maryland: Aspen Publishers, 1(1):1–8, 1986.

9. Rudolf J: Automated gastric lavage and a comparison of 0.9% normal saline solution and tap water irrigant. *Ann Emerg Med* 14:1156–1159, 1985.

10. Goodman CS, Gilman A: The pharmacologic basis of therapeutics. New York: Macmillan, 1986.

11. Manogurra AS: Tricyclic antidepressants. *Crit Care Q* 5(4):43–52, 1982.

12. Marshall JB, Forker AD: Cardiovascular effects of TCA drugs, therapeutic usage, overdose and management of complications. *Am Heart J* 103:401–414, 1982.

13. Pental P, Sioris L: Incidence of late arrhythmia following TCA overdose. *Clin Toxicol* 18:543–548, 1981.

14. Hagerman G, Hanashiro P: Reversal of tricyclic antidepressant-induced cardiac conduction abnormalities by phenytoin. *Ann Emerg Med* 10:82–86, 1980.

15. Callaham M: Epidemiology of fatal tricyclic antidepressant ingestion: Implications for management. *Ann Emerg Med* 14:29–37, 1985.

CHAPTER 2
Cardiovascular Health System

Overview

The cardiovascular health system is concerned with the supply of blood to the body tissues through the heart and blood vessels. Many patients present with either primary or secondary alterations in health status in this system. Alterations in cardiovascular status most frequently determine the patient's level of acuity and need for timely intervention regardless of presenting complaint.

Case studies selected for this section discuss patients with an alteration in red blood cells (sickle cell crisis) and with myocardial events (ischemia, infarction, and tachydysrhythmia). Other patients who present with alterations in the cardiovascular health system but are not included in this grouping of studies include patients with peripheral vascular occlusion or disease, bleeding disorders such as hemophilia, high blood pressure, dyspnea on exertion or activity intolerance, and acute hemorrhages such as GI bleeding.

CUE WORDS ▬▬▬▬▬▬▬▬

BLOOD
bleeding
clotting
erythrocytes
plasma
platelets
volume

CARDIOVASCULAR
activity tolerance
cardiac output
heart
peripheral circulation
tissue perfusion
vessels

RELATED NURSING DIAGNOSES ▬▬▬▬▬▬▬

activity intolerance
fatigue
potential activity intolerance
decreased cardiac output
fluid volume excess
fluid volume deficit
potential fluid volume deficit
altered tissue perfusion (specify)

Department of Emergency Medicine Triage Protocols

Cardiovascular Health System

Level I	Level II	Level III	Level IV
Chest pain, nonradiating; less than 30 years old; no personal or family hx of cardiac disease; VSS; no associated cardiac symptoms; diaphoresis, N/V, SOB, pallor	Chest pain, continuous, sharp, increases with movement; associated with cough; no SOB	Chest pain, relieved by NTG; hx angina or cardiac disease; no current chest pain	Chest pain, sudden onset; diaphoresis, nausea, pallor; may or may not have cardiac hx
		hx heart disease; peripheral edema noted; 60 < HR < 120; c/o SOB on exertion, not currently SOB	Pacemaker dependent, c/o weakness, syncope;
			Pulse rate more than 150 or less than 45;
			Irregular pulse rate, rapid, new onset; symptomatic patient: weak, dizzy, hypotensive, impaired mentation, recent syncopal episode
Bleeding disorder; presents for elective transfusion; asymptomatic		Bleeding disorder, presents with (a) joint pain and/or swelling, (b) hx trauma, (c) presents for cryotherapy	Bleeding disorder, overt bleeding, signs of bleeding into joints, etc.

Wants BP check, entrance into clinic system	Sickle cell patients experiencing mild to moderate pain; afebrile; no nausea or vomiting	Sickle cell patients now having moderate to severe pain; may be febrile; nausea and vomiting	Sickle cell crisis, severe pain, symptoms of ischemia, hypoxia, respiratory distress
	Hypertensive, ran out of medication, in no acute distress; systolic < 200, diastolic < 115	Hypertensive, headache, no neurological deficit; diastolic 115–130	Hypertensive crisis, diastolic > 130; hypertensive with weakness, chest pain, neurological deficits
	Hypotensive; not symptomatic	Hypotensive secondary to volume deficit; orthostatic changes	Hypotensive, shocky, unstable
		Leg pain with decreased circulation, decreased sensation; calf pain; warm erythematous, edematous leg; positive Homan's sign	Pulseless, cold, cyanotic extremity; or same as III plus SOB

2.1 SICKLE CELL ANEMIA: WHEN IT'S A CRISIS
Kathleen A. Williams, RN, BSN

H.C. is a 28-year-old black male with sickle cell anemia. He is well known to the ED staff and has visited the emergency room 3 times over the past week. He has had six visits over the past month. The precipitating cause for H.C.'s previous six visits appears to have been an upper respiratory infection. He has been experiencing a productive cough and low-grade fever both of which have resolved with antibiotic therapy. On H.C.'s most recent visit, 2 days ago, he described his usual crisis pain involving both knees, right hip, and back. His pain resolved with two morphine injections over a 5-hr period. He was able to tolerate oral rehydration and was discharged with a prescription for oral pain medication. Attempts to manage his pain at home with oral analgesics and fluids have been unsuccessful. He presently rates his pain as a 9 on a scale of 1 to 10. He has been experiencing intermittent nausea and vomiting.

H.C.'s previous history includes a seizure disorder due to a cerebral infarction at age 21 and a splenectomy due to a sickle cell sequestration event at age 14. H.C. denies any drug or alcohol abuse.

Triage Assessment, Acuity Level III: Sickle cell patient with moderate to severe pain.

Within 15 min H.C. is brought to the treatment area for further examination and intervention. On exam, H.C. appears to be in moderate to severe distress, rocking in pain on the stretcher. He is alert and oriented, pupils equal and reactive, conjunctiva pale, sclerae mildly icteric. Lung fields are clear to auscultation. Cardiac assessment is within normal limits. H.C.'s abdomen is soft and nontender with active bowel sounds. His extremities are without edema, cyanosis, pallor, or clubbing. His distal pulses are present in all limbs. No priapism is observed.

H.C. denies any recent trauma to his knees, hip, or back. No deformities can be palpated, although each area is tender to touch. His orthostatic vital signs are lying BP 170/98, pulse 88, respirations 22; and standing BP 140/104 and pulse 120. Rectal temperature is 99.4° F. The labs ordered by the physician have the following results: hematocrit 22.8, white-blood-cell (WBC) count 12.1, reticulocytes 12.1, sodium 140, potassium 4.5, chloride 111, CO_2 20, urea nitrogen 9, creatinine 1.7, glucose 82, total bilirubin 4.0, amylase 67, and magnesium 1.5. These results are not significantly different from H.C.'s lab results obtained during his visit 2 days prior.

After consultation with the doctor, H.C. is medicated by the nurse with 8 mg morphine sulfate intramuscularly. Heating pads and pillows are applied to his knees and back. Because of his inability to tolerate oral fluids, an intravenous solution of 5% dextrose and 0.45% normal saline is started at 150 ml/hr. After 6 hr, H.C.'s vital signs are normal with intravenous rehydration. However, he is still unable to tolerate oral fluids and he has received two additional intramuscular morphine sulfate injections without significant management of his pain. A decision is made by the physician to admit H.C. to the hospital with a diagnosis of vaso-occlusive sickle cell crisis.

QUESTIONS AND ANSWERS

1. **What is a sickle cell crisis?**

   Sickle cell anemia (SCA) is an autosomal recessive disease. This homozygotic state afflicts 1 in every 500 blacks in the United States (1). The heterozygotic state of carrying the sickle cell trait is benign under normal conditions but is important from a genetic standpoint. If two individuals carrying the sickle cell trait mate, their children would have a one in four chance of having SCA (1). Therefore, patients with sickle cell trait need appropriate genetic and family planning counseling.

   SCA is caused by abnormalities in the hemoglobin structure of red blood cells. The abnormalities are caused by substitutions that occur in the two amino acid chains which form hemoglobin (Hb). This substitution causes the "sickling" of erythrocytes under certain conditions. Red blood cells from patients with SCA contain 80 to 100% of the abnormal Hb chain known as HbS. Patients with sickle cell trait contain 20 to 45% HbS (1).

   Decreased oxygen tension will induce a sickling episode, also known as a sickle cell crisis (SCC). Events which may contribute to a decrease in O_2 tension include anesthesia (by causing a transient episode of hypoxia), exercise, infection, acidosis, and dehydration (1). During periods of decreased oxygen tension the solubility of HbS is decreased due to the "sickling" or clumping of Hb. The sickled red blood cell becomes very rigid and can assume dramatic changes in shape. This change in shape will decrease the available surface area for oxygen transport. Small vessels can become partially or completely occluded by these rigid, sickled, erythrocytes. This occlusion of the blood vessel will cause ischemia, pain, infarction, and dysfunction of the tissue distal to the occlusion (1).

   Certain organ systems are particularly susceptible to dysfunction due to SCA. These include organs where blood flow is slow and highly vascular such as the spleen, liver, and renal medulla. The brain, muscle tissue, and maternal placenta are also at risk for infarction due to SCA because of high metabolic demand (1).

2. **What are the types of SCCs, and which type is H.C. experiencing?**

   Generally, there are four types of SCCs.

   Sequestration is usually seen in children and is caused by blood pooling in the abdominal viscera as the result of a sickling episode. This pooling of blood will cause a dramatic drop in the patient's hematocrit and may be fatal. The organ usually involved in the sickling episode is the spleen. Often sickle cell patients have had a splenectomy as a child or adolescent due to a sequestration episode. The spleen may also infarct due to a sequestration episode leading to fibrosis and atrophy of the spleen (1–3).

Aplastic crisis is due to a temporary cessation of erythropoiesis. This usually follows an infection. The patient's blood count and reticulocyte count need to be followed closely to determine that the patient has regained the ability to produce red blood cells. An aplastic crisis is usually self-limiting (3, 4).

Hemolytic crisis is manifested by a drop in Hb due to a rapid increase in hemolysis. A patient will have an increased reticulocyte count as the body attempts to compensate by increasing erythropoiesis. These patients will have a decreased hematocrit and elevated bilirubin. This type of crisis is rare and may be associated with a concomitant deficiency of the enzyme glucose-6-phosphate dehydrogenase (G6PD). This enzyme deficiency is also prevalent in the black population in general (1–3).

Occlusive crisis is caused by ischemia or infarction from vascular occlusion. A vaso-occlusive crisis may occur anywhere in the body but is common in long bones, joints, and the spine. Abdominal pain from an occlusive crisis must be differentiated from an acute surgical abdomen. An occlusive crisis may lead to a cerebral vascular accident, kidney infarction, lung infarction, bone necrosis, and priapism (1, 2).

H.C.'s crisis would be described as a vaso-occlusive crisis in his knees, hip, and back, supported by his physical exam, labs, and history. His abdominal exam is benign, so he is not having a sequestration crisis. H.C.'s hematocrit, hemoglobin, and bilirubin are at baseline which rules out a hemolytic or aplastic crisis.

TIP: SCA is associated with a partially compensated hemolytic anemia. Red blood cells in SCA patients have a shorter life span. Red blood cells which have sickled will hemolyze due to structural damage to the cell and stasis in areas of diminished circulation. This is the pathophysiological reason for H.C. to have chronic anemia and hyperbilirubinemia (1).

---

3. **What are the nursing diagnoses appropriate for H.C.?**
    Diagnosis: Pain related to ischemia of joints and bones caused by SCA
        Desired patient outcome: The patient will state that his pain has been relieved to a level he can manage at home on oral analgesics.
    Diagnosis: Fluid volume deficit related to inadequate fluid intake, nausea, and vomiting

<u>Desired patient outcome:</u> The patient will receive adequate intravenous hydration demonstrated by nonorthostatic vital signs and will tolerate oral liquids.

Diagnosis: Altered peripheral tissue perfusion related to decreased oxygen tension and transport to bones and joints caused by SCA

<u>Desired patient outcome:</u> The patient will have adequate tissue perfusion demonstrated by fewer complaints of pain, adequate urinary output (> 30 ml/hr), and capillary refill less than 2 sec.

Diagnosis: Anxiety related to chronicity of illness, pain, and frequency of ED visits

<u>Desired patient outcome:</u> H.C. will verbalize his feelings regarding his ED visit and remain actively involved in his care and management. He will state two coping strategies to manage his pain at home.

4. **What are the nursing interventions related to H.C.'s nursing diagnoses?**

All patients presenting to the ED need a baseline set of vital signs, a physical assessment, and a pain assessment. The physical exam was presented earlier. It is important to look for other potential medical and surgical causes besides SCC. For example a patient complaining of abdominal pain may have an acute surgical abdomen. The nurse needs to keep a high index of suspicion for other potential problems with this patient population (5).

An initial and ongoing assessment of the patient's pain level will assist in the evaluation of nursing and medical interventions. The acronym PQRST is useful in pain assessment (5).

P: Provocation—what brought about this episode?
Q: Quality—is there anything different about this episode?
R: Region—is this the usual area of your SSC?
S: Severity—what rating would you give your pain on a scale from 1 to 10?
T: Time—how long have you had this pain?

To manage the patient's pain the nurse should provide increased fluid intake, orally if possible. The patient should be encouraged to drink juices, soda, or an electrolyte solution such as Pedialyte. Intravenous fluids are recommended to be started only if the patient is unable to take fluids orally. This preserves venous access (5).

TIP: Because of the renal sequelae of SCC, many SCA patients are unable to concentrate their urine. Therefore, water will not adequately rehydrate them. This inability to concentrate their urine can precipitate a vaso-occlusive crisis. The usual fluid requirement of a SCA patient is 3 to 5 liters per day (6). That's 250 to 400 ml per waking hour.

The nurse should monitor and record intake and output, orthostatic vital signs, and skin turgor to reassess hydration. The nurse should assess for fluid overload in older patients through frequent auscultation of the patient's lung fluids (6). Comfort measures should be provided such as pillows under joints, and heating pads. Distraction or diversional activities may also help break the pain cycle. Analgesics should be administered as ordered.

TIP: Meperidine is contraindicated with SCA patients who have known seizure disorders because it lowers the seizure threshold even with therapeutic anticonvulsant medication levels (6).

A physical assessment and pain assessment should be performed within 1 hr after each dose of medication to evaluate the patient's response. The patient should be allowed to control his pain management as much as possible including dose and frequency of medication based on his known baseline, and preferred site of administration. Persistent pain, unrelieved by medication and other measures described may indicate a more serious vasoocclusive event. Although pain is always difficult to evaluate, it should not be assumed that the patient's presentation is related to drug-seeking behavior. A sickle cell crisis is real. The patient may have reached some tolerance level for the medications being prescribed necessitating more than the usual dosage and frequency. The nurse should work with the patient and the doctor to identify alternate medications or medication combinations to help relieve the pain. As with the pain associated with an acute myocardial infarction, the pain of SSC should be relieved as quickly as possible.

TIP: The patient should be encouraged to rest or lie quietly on the stretcher. "Rocking" in pain can increase the metabolic and oxygen demands of the affected tissue by 75% and exacerbate the crisis situation (4).

The nurse's role in managing H.C.'s altered tissue perfusion includes monitoring the patient for signs of increasing pain, decreased urinary output, and clinical presentation of shocklike symptoms.

5. How would the nurse evaluate H.C.'s care?

Because H.C. was not achieving the desired patient outcomes after 6 hr of definitive care, the physician, in collaboration with the nurse, decided that more aggressive therapy was needed including admission to the hospital. H.C. was scheduled for a CT scan of his hip to rule out infarction and plans were made for continuous intravenous morphine infusion to provide for more adequate pain control. In preparing the patient for admission to the hospital the nurse gave a report to the inpatient unit nurse describing the nursing problems identified, H.C.'s usual coping strategies, and the status of the current desired outcomes.

REFERENCES

1. Management and treatment of sickle cell disease. U.S. Department of Health and Human Services *NIH publication*, Sept. 1984.

2. Charache S: Treatment of sickle cell anemia. *Annu Rev Med* 32:195–206, 1981.

3. Barnhart M, Henry R, Lusher J: Sickle Cell. Kalamazoo, Michigan: Upjohn Co., 1976.

4. Charache S: Management of patients with sickle cell anemia in the E.R. Baltimore: Johns Hopkins Hospital Department of Medicine. *Sickle Cell Protocol*, 1986.

5. Bourg P, Sherer C, Rosen P: Standardized nursing care plans for the emergency department. St. Louis: C. V. Mosby, 166–169, 1986.

6. The Nurses' Reference Library. Emergencies. Springhouse, Pennsylvania: Springhouse Corp., 480, 1985.

2.2 ACUTE MYOCARDIAL INFARCTION: THROMBOLYTIC THERAPY IN THE EMERGENCY DEPARTMENT

Valerie A. Barron, RN, BSN, CCRN, CEN

Jason R. is a 38-year-old white male who called the ED about 30 min prior to arrival to ask if he should come to the hospital. Jason said over the phone, "My wife's bugging me to come over there. I've got a heavy pressure in my chest, sort of like indigestion. I've had it before, but it always went away. This time I can't get rid of it." Jason was advised by the ED nurse to come to the hospital, preferably by ambulance.

Jason arrived by car and is noted to look pale and uncomfortable. He complains of pain in the center of his chest that feels like a heavy pressure that is now going down both arms. The pain has increased in severity since he left home. Jason rates his pain as 8 on a scale of 1 to 10. Jason is assisted to a stretcher and while lying in semi-Fowler's position has no dyspnea. His vital signs are temperature 99°F, pulse 60 and regular, respiratory rate 22, and BP 108/60. Lung sounds are clear and heart sounds are regular with normal S1 and S2. He has an extra heart sound, S4.

When questioned about recent health, Jason tells the nurse that he has had chest pain off and on for about 1 week. Jason describes the pain as a tightness or heaviness in the center of his chest under the breastbone. Jason also mentions that the pain occurs with physical exertion and goes away with rest.

Jason is married and has two children. He is a sales executive and received a promotion 1 month ago. Jason smokes about one pack of cigarettes per day. He has no previous medical history and does not take any drugs. Jason says that his father died of a heart attack and his mother has hypertension.

Triage Assessment, Acuity Level IV: Chest pain, unrelieved; pain continues at rest.

Jason is taken immediately to the treatment area to rule out myocardial ischemia or injury. A 12-lead ECG is immediately done and reveals ST segment elevation in leads I, II, III, AVF, V4, V5, and V6. T waves are inverted in V1, V2, and V3, and an abnormal R wave is present in V1. The initial creatine phosphokinase (CPK) is reported as 153 (0 to 225 is normal). The ED physician makes a diagnosis of acute inferior lateral myocardial infarction (MI). True posterior MI is also considered.

Jason is given oxygen via nasal cannula at 5 liters/min and sublingual nitroglycerin with significant reduction in his pain. After consultation with a cardiologist, Jason is deemed a candidate for thrombolytic therapy. A lidocaine bolus is administered per protocol and a continuous infusion of lidocaine is started at 2 mg/min. Tissue plasminogen activator (t-PA) is selected as the thrombolytic agent for Jason. An intravenous bolus dose of 10 mg of t-PA is given by the physician, and an infusion of t-PA is initiated at a rate of 50 mg/hr. Jason is then transferred to the coronary care unit (CCU) for further definitive therapy and monitoring.

QUESTIONS AND ANSWERS

1. **What is the significance of the risk factors for coronary heart disease that can be identified for Jason?**

   Although the mortality rate for cardiovascular disease has decreased from 39% in 1964 to 19% in 1984, 60% of the deaths related to myocardial infarction occur outside the hospital (1). Prevention of sudden death due to acute myocardial infarction (AMI) can be enhanced through efforts directed at early recognition of symptoms and risk factors. Risk factors identified for Jason include sex (incidence of AMI occurs more often in men than in premenopausal women), cigarette smoking (associated with an AMI risk 2.5 times greater than nonsmokers), and family history positive for coronary heart disease (1).

   In addition, Jason seems to have experienced a recent increase in stress, related to his job promotion. Stress, hypertension, diabetes mellitus, and elevated cholesterol are all risk factors for CHD and occurrence of AMI.

   Chest pain should also be recognized as a risk factor. The importance of the patient acknowledging chest pain as a potential precursor of sudden death is essential in order to reduce prehospital mortality from CHD. Educational efforts by the American Heart Association

(AHA) emphasize the importance of not only recognizing risk factors, but also the importance of seeking medical intervention at the onset of symptoms. In particular, the role of the spouse or significant other is stressed; this person might encourage their loved one to seek medical attention when he or she has chest pain. Jason had chest pain for about a week before his AMI. He was reluctant to come to the hospital and called for advice only at the urging of his wife. Educational efforts need to continue to alert people like Jason to request medical help as soon as they experience chest pain.

2. **How does the progression of coronary artery disease relate to current theories about the pathophysiology of AMI?**

   The pathogenesis of coronary artery disease involves a progressive narrowing of the lumen of the coronary artery. The coronary arteries become stenotic due to an increase in the formation of plaque in the vessels. These narrowed coronary vessels give rise to the formation of thrombi.

   A recent investigation of the pathophysiology of AMI demonstrated that in 80 to 90% of cases of transmural MI (through the entire thickness of the myocardium), coronary artery thrombosis was identified as the causative factor (2). Thrombus formation results in complete occlusion of the coronary artery. As blood flow and oxygen are drastically reduced to the myocardium, necrosis occurs. Research findings indicate that the process of myocardial necrosis is complete after about 6 hr (2).

3. **How is the diagnosis of AMI determined?**

   Three criteria are important for the diagnosis of AMI: clinical presentation, ECG findings, and cardiac enzyme studies. The most significant component is the clinical picture. If a person presents with symptoms of AMI, appropriate medical evaluation and treatment should be initiated even if the ECG and/or cardiac enzymes are normal.

TIP: Careful analysis of a patient's complaint of chest pain is critical in order to develop the plan of nursing care. Use the following mnemonic to assist with collection of assessment data: PQRST (Fig. 2.2.1).

If the chest pain is associated with dyspnea, dizziness, weakness, or diaphoresis, the patient should be observed with cardiac monitoring and have further diagnostic evaluation. If ECG changes of ischemia, injury, or infarction (necrosis) are present and the patient has chest pain, the diagnosis of CHD is fairly certain.

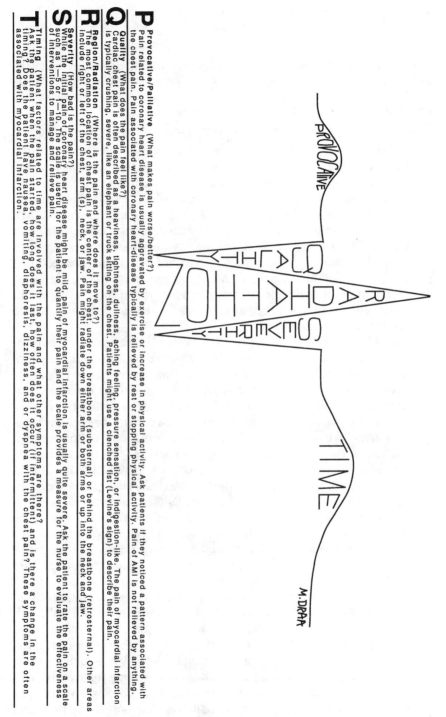

P **Provocative/Palliative** (What makes pain worse/better?)
Pain related to coronary heart disease is usually aggravated by exercise or increase in physical activity. Ask patients if they noticed a pattern associated with the chest pain. Pain associated with coronary heart-disease typically is relieved by rest or stopping physical activity. Pain of AMI is not relieved by anything.

Q **Quality** (What does the pain feel like?)
Cardiac chest pain is often described as a heaviness, tightness, dullness, aching feeling, pressure sensation, or indigestion-like. The pain of myocardial infarction is typically crushing, severe, like an elephant or truck sitting on the chest. Patients might use a clenched fist (Levine's sign) to describe their pain.

R **Region/Radiation** (Where is the pain and where does it move to?)
The most common location of chest pain is the center of the chest; under the breastbone (substernal) or behind the breastbone (retrosternal). Other areas include right or left of the chest, arm (s), neck, or jaw. Pain might radiate down either arm or both arms or up into the neck and jaw.

S **Severity** (How bad is the pain?)
While the initial pain of coronary heart disease might be mild, pain of myocardial infarction is usually quite severe. Ask the patient to rate the pain on a scale such as 1—5 or 1—10. The scale is useful for the patient to quantify their pain and the scale provides a measure for the nurse to evaluate the effectiveness of interventions to manage and relieve pain.

T **Timing** (What factors related to time are involved with the pain and what other symptoms are there?
Ask the patient when the pain started, how long does it last, how often does it occur (if intermittent) and is there a change in the timing? Does the patient have nausea, vomiting, diaphoresis, dizziness, and or dyspnea with the chest pain? These symptoms are often associated with myocardial infarction.

Figure 2.2.1. Assessment of chest pain. (Illustration by Marsha A. Draa, RN.)

TIP: A normal ECG does not rule out the diagnosis of CHD or even myocardial infarction. Initial ECG tracings may be normal in patients with AMI or angina. The 12-lead ECG should be repeated at periodic intervals, when a change in patient status occurs, and when the pattern of chest pain changes.

The 12-lead ECG can show changes associated with myocardial ischemia, injury, or infarction (Fig. 2.2.2), and these changes can occur without symptoms. For example, the patient with diabetes mellitus and related neuropathy might have a "silent" MI. In this situation the patient reports little or no chest pain, but the ECG shows AMI. This patient might present to the ED with new onset congestive heart failure (CHF). Another example involves the patient who experiences "silent" ischemia. ECG changes of myocardial ischemia are recorded during routine monitoring of an asymptomatic patient, via 24-hr Holter or ambulatory monitoring (3). This type of monitoring might be done for people who are at high risk for developing CHD but do not yet have symptoms.

ECG changes may be present only when the patient complains of chest pain, indicative of variant or Prinzmetal's angina (4). This atypical form of angina is not precipitated by factors of physical or emotional stress usually associated with angina. The symptoms occur without warning and are often short-lived. The etiology of variant angina is coronary artery spasm. When a spasm occurs in a coronary vessel, the coronary artery is temporarily occluded. The flow of blood and oxygen to a portion of the myocardium is severely restricted. At this time ECG changes of ischemia and injury are seen. When the vessel relaxes, blood flow is reestablished, and the symptoms and ECG change disappear. Serial recordings of the ECG are useful under these circumstances.

If an ECG shows any change initially, subsequent tracings can be used to evaluate patient progress. This is particularly important for the patient who receives thrombolytic therapy. If the occluded vessel is opened by the thrombolytic drug, the ECG should show resolution of the initial ischemia or injury pattern.

Various ECG leads record different surfaces of the myocardium. Leads II, III, and AVF record the inferior portion; leads I, AVL, V5, and V6 record the lateral surface; and VI through V4 reflect the anterior septal area. There is no direct lead to record the posterior surface, but changes in VI will show an abnormally tall R wave (sometimes referred to as a mirror image). ECG changes indicating right ventricular infarction can be seen with right ventricular leads. Right ventricular leads are recorded from the right side of the chest using the same landmarks as the standard precordial leads.

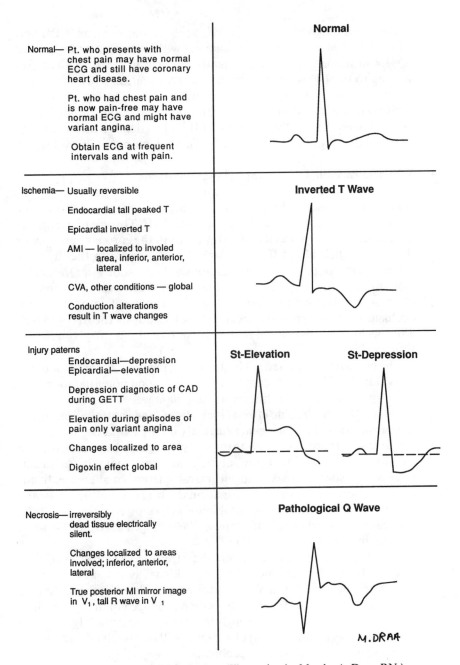

Normal— Pt. who presents with chest pain may have normal ECG and still have coronary heart disease.

Pt. who had chest pain and is now pain-free may have normal ECG and might have variant angina.

Obtain ECG at frequent intervals and with pain.

Normal

Ischemia— Usually reversible

Endocardial tall peaked T

Epicardial inverted T

AMI — localized to involed area, inferior, anterior, lateral

CVA, other conditions — global

Conduction alterations result in T wave changes

Inverted T Wave

Injury paterns
Endocardial—depression
Epicardial—elevation

Depression diagnostic of CAD during GETT

Elevation during episodes of pain only variant angina

Changes localized to area

Digoxin effect global

St-Elevation   **St-Depression**

Necrosis— irreversibly dead tissue electrically silent.

Changes localized to areas involved; inferior, anterior, lateral

True posterior MI mirror image in V_1, tall R wave in V_1

Pathological Q Wave

M.DRAA

Figure 2.2.2. Lead ECG changes. (Illustration by Marsha A. Draa, RN.)

The third diagnostic tool of AMI is the cardiac enzyme. CPK and CPK MB isoenzymes will show changes within the first 4 to 6 hr after AMI. Cardiac enzymes are frequently not helpful for the patient presenting to the ED with chest pain of short duration since the values obtained from the initial sample drawn in the ED may be normal. However, the decision to use thrombolytic therapy cannot be delayed. Therefore, the diagnosis of AMI will be determined by the patient's clinical presentation and ECG, as demonstrated by Jason's case.

4. **Why was thrombolytic therapy chosen for Jason?**

Thrombolytic therapy is the administration of pharmacological agents that dissolve blood clots. As mentioned above, coronary thrombosis is recognized as the etiology of AMI. Thrombolytic agents are administered to dissolve the thrombus in the coronary artery and thus reestablish blood flow through the vessel and to the myocardium. If the blood flow can be reestablished very soon after the occlusion, myocardial necrosis can be prevented. The onset of symptoms of chest pain is generally correlated with the onset of coronary artery occlusion. Since myocardial necrosis evolves during the first 4 to 6 hr after occlusion, it is critical that thrombolytic drugs are given in this time period.

The chest pain experienced by Jason began about 2.5 hr prior to his arrival in the ED. This meant that there was good potential for reversal or minimalization of his myocardial damage.

5. **What are the effects, side effects, indications, and contraindications of the various thrombolytic agents currently on the market?**

Currently there are three thrombolytic agents available for the treatment of AMI. The thrombolytic drugs are streptokinase, urokinase, and tissue type plasminogen activator (t-PA) or alteplase. In addition, there are two investigational drugs in clinical trials: anisoylated plasminogen-streptokinase activator complex (ASPAC, eminase) and single-chain urokinase plasminogen activator (scu-PA, prourokinase) (5).

Streptokinase is derived from the streptococcal bacteria. The thrombolytic effect produced by streptokinase is systemic since the drug combines with circulating plasminogen. Plasmin, the substance that actually dissolves fibrin clots, is then produced in the circulation. As the plasmin circulates through the body, a systemic "lytic" state develops. This means that all blood clots will be dissolved and the patient might develop bleeding problems.

Other problems associated with streptokinase are the prolonged effect on the coagulation system (18 to 24 hr after the drug is given), hypotension associated with administration of the drug, and the possibility of allergic reactions to this "foreign" substance and of resistance to the drug because of patient antibodies to streptococcus bacteria (6). Major contraindications to the use of streptokinase are recent strep infections, recent intracranial or intraspinal surgery or trauma, intracranial aneurysm, neoplasm or arteriovenous malformation, history of cerebrovascular accident (CVA), active internal bleeding, uncontrolled hypertension, or known bleeding tendency or disorder.

Urokinase is a naturally occurring human enzyme, found in small amounts in urine and produced by kidney cells. Urokinase converts plasminogen to plasmin in the circulation and produces a systemic lytic state much the same as the effects of streptokinase. Since urokinase is a natural substance, there is less chance of allergic reactions and hypotension.

Tissue plasminogen activator is a natural substance found in blood cells. It is referred to as a clot-specific or clot-selective drug since it binds with fibrin at the site of the newly formed blood clot. This binding results in the conversion of plasminogen at the site of the clot to plasmin. The effects of t-PA then are limited to specific fresh blood clots. Side effects are minimal—bleeding from fresh blood clots might occur. Major contraindications to t-PA are similar to those for other thrombolytic agents. Other possible contraindications include surgery within the last 10 days, cerebrovascular disease, hypertension, pregnancy, and any other conditions in which the risk of bleeding is great. Patients must be evaluated individually on a risk/benefit basis.

The investigational drugs previously mentioned are modified versions of the originals. These drugs, like t-PA, are designed to be clot-specific and do not result in systemic lytic states.

6. **What are the specific nursing care concerns related to patients receiving t-PA?**

The first concern of the nurse is to assist in the identification of patients who might be candidates for t-PA or any thrombolytic therapy. Patients presenting with chest pain must be carefully screened and evaluated according to the above criteria. If the nurse suspects that the patient might be a candidate for thrombolytic therapy, blood samples should be obtained for coagulation studies along with the other initial blood work. Blood samples should be obtained through an intravenous catheter with a heparin lock adapter to prevent open venipuncture sites. If venipuncture is attempted and missed, a pressure dressing should be applied and the site clearly identified. Generally three intravenous sites will be needed.

If the thrombolytic agent is not readily available in the ED, the pharmacy should be notified as soon as possible. It is imperative that the drug be administered within 6 hr after the onset of the patient's chest pain. It should be noted that thrombolytic agents are very expensive and should be handled carefully. If t-PA is the agent selected, the intravenous bolus dose should be prepared for the physician to administer and then the intravenous infusion immediately started. Intravenous infusion devices must be used to ensure the accuracy of the drug administration. Protocols may vary by hospital, but the usual dose of t-PA is 100 mg within 6 hr: an initial bolus of 6 to 10 mg followed by 50 mg administered by infusion over the first hour and 40 mg by continuous infusion over the next 2 to 5 hr.

While hypotension is usually not associated with t-PA, the patient requires close monitoring of vital signs during drug administration. Continuous cardiac monitoring will help to identify reperfusion when it occurs. During reperfusion of the myocardium (if t-PA has dissolved the clot and reestablished blood flow through the coronary vessel), a variety of dysrhythmias will be noted on the monitor. These dysrhythmias occur due to reestablishment of blood flow to a hypoxic myocardium, making cells irritable and capable of chaotic electrical impulse formation.

7. **What nursing diagnoses can be determined for Jason?**

The following nursing diagnoses are appropriate for Jason.

Diagnosis: Potential for decreased cardiac output related to development of lethal dysrhythmias as evidenced by premature ventricular contractions (PVCs), ventricular tachycardia, (VT), and ventricular fibrillation (VF)

Desired patient outcome: The patient maintains a normal sinus rhythm, systolic BP > 90 mm Hg, and urinary output > 30 ml/hr; the patient remains alert and oriented.

Diagnosis: Altered coronary tissue perfusion related to decreased coronary artery blood flow as evidenced by chest pain and by ischemia or injury pattern on 12-lead ECG

Desired patient outcome: The patient states that there is a decrease in and/or relief of chest pain, and 12-lead ECG shows return to baseline or normal.

Diagnosis: Anxiety related to hospitalization and potential for death as evidenced by facial tension, restlessness, and questions asked by patient

Desired patient outcome: The patient will demonstrate reduction of anxiety by relaxed facial muscles and ability to rest; the patient will describe his feelings and demonstrate coping strategies that reduce feelings of anxiety.

Diagnosis: Potential for injury related to complications of thrombolytic therapy such as bruising and bleeding

Desired patient outcome: The patient will have no evidence of bleeding and minimal bruising.

Diagnosis: Potential ineffective family coping related to onset of critical illness as evidenced by wife's questions and interaction with patient

Desired patient outcome: Wife of patient will verbalize understanding of husband's condition and support system needs. The patient and his wife will state strategies for assisting each other through this illness; the patient and his wife will state other resources available such as other supportive family members.

8. **What are the nursing interventions necessary to manage the care of Jason?**

Prompt attention to the first two nursing diagnoses takes priority since these diagnoses involve potentially life-threatening conditions. The nurse should obtain a history of the patient's chest pain and risk factors for CHD. The patient should be assisted with lying down on a stretcher, in a comfortable position. Rest and comfortable body position can help to decrease myocardial oxygen demands. The 12-lead ECG should be recorded quickly and cardiac monitoring initiated at once. This will allow for quick detection of potentially life-threatening dysrhythmias. Myocardial ischemia, injury, or necrosis should also be quickly identified.

Since all patients with cardiac chest pain (or chest pain with undetermined etiology) are possible candidates for thrombolytic therapy, care must be taken with venipuncture as previously described. Blood samples should be sent for cardiac enzymes (including MB isoenzymes), coagulation studies, CBC, blood urea nitrogen (BUN), glucose, and electrolytes.

Oxygen is administered via nasal cannula at 3 to 5 liters/min. If the patient is known to have chronic obstructive pulmonary disease and has a tendency to retain CO_2, oxygen should be given at 2 to 3 liters/min. It is important to increase the amount of circulating oxygen to the myocardium. Reassurance and explanations about the hospital routines help to decrease anxiety and therefore myocardial oxygen demands.

Chest pain management is directed at efforts to enhance coronary blood flow. Medications of choice include nitroglycerin (sublingual, oral, topical, or intravenous); calcium channel blockers such as nifedipine; and analgesics such as morphine and meperidine. Beta-blockers might also be administered to decrease myocardial oxygen demands. Patient response to these cardiovascular medications should be monitored closely by the nurse. Frequent evaluation of chest pain and vital signs is essential. Medications are usually titrated to control chest pain as long as vital signs are stable. Communication with family and/or significant others is important in terms of aiding the family as well as patient coping. The family should be allowed to see the patient as soon as reasonably possible. Patients may benefit from familiar support systems as they make crucial decisions about their care (for example, thrombolytic therapy or choosing a physician). In addition, family members should be encouraged to call upon their own support systems. AMI is a life-threatening illness. Spiritual support should be offered and provided as requested by the patient or family member.

Emergency equipment, defibrillator, medications, airway, and ambu bag should be kept at the bedside and transported with the patient. The staff should be prepared to treat sudden cardiac arrest at any time.

The patient who comes to the ED with chest pain is usually very anxious. The notion of a heart attack is feared by the patient. Fears associated with a heart attack include fear of death and disability. Many patients fear that if they do survive, their lives will never be the same. The nurse must respond to the patient's verbal and nonverbal concerns. Honest, clear explanations should be provided for the patient and family. Concrete terminology should be used to explain what will happen to the patient. Explanations provided by the ED nurse will include a description of the CCU and the admission procedures. When the patient is transferred to the CCU, the ED nurse should accompany him and introduce him to the CCU nursing staff (7), provide a complete report, and update the nursing care plan based on the patient's response to treatment.

REFERENCES

1. American Heart Association. Textbook of advanced cardiac life support. Dallas, Texas, 1987.
2. Misinski M: Pathophysiology of acute myocardial infarction: A rationale for thrombolytic therapy [Part 2 supplement]. *Heart Lung* 17 (6):743–750, 1988.
3. Assey ME: Ischemia without symptoms. *Emerg Med* 20 (7):26–36, 1988.
4. Schakenback LH: Prinzmetal's angina: Current perceptions and treatments. *Crit Care Nurse* (2):90–99, 1987.

5. Kleven MR: Comparison of thrombolytic agents: Mechanism of action, efficacy, and safety [Part 2 supplement]. *Heart Lung* 17(6):750–755, 1988.

6. Henderson E: Clinical experience with thrombolytic agents [Part 2]. *J Emerg Nur* 15(2):174–181, 1989.

7. Throwe AN, Fought SG: Psychosocial nursing care of the emergency patient. New York: John Wiley & Sons, 1984.

SUGGESTED READINGS

Belle-Isle C: Patient selection and administration of thrombolytic therapy; Part 2. *J Emerg Nurs* 15(2):155–162, 1989.
Conover M: Electrocardiography update: 1988. *J Cardiovasc Nurs* 2(4):45–52, 1988.
Dracup KA, Weinberg SL, eds: Symposium proceedings: Nursing interventions in

limiting infarct size in acute MI patient. *Heart Lung* 16(6) (suppl): 739–800, 1988.

Erickson DE, Kleven M: Patient care guidelines, the acute myocardial infarction patient receiving tissue-type plasminogen activator. *J Emerg Nurs* 14(4):253–259, 1988.

Giebl RA, Pavey SS, Bryant PP: t-PA therapy in acute myocardial infarction. *J Emerg Nurs* 14(4);253–259, 1988.

Gillis CL, Sparancino PSA, Gortner SR, Kenneth HY: Events leading to the treatment of coronary artery disease: Implications for nursing care. *Heart Lung* 14(4):350–356, 1985.

Funk M: Diagnosis of right ventricular infarction with right precordial leads. *Heart Lung* 15(6):562–570, 1986.

Henderson E: Thrombolytic therapy in acute myocardial infarction: An overview [Part 2]. *J Emerg Nurs* 15(2):145–149, 1989.

Lee TH, Rouan GW, Weisberg ME, et al.: Clinical characteristics and natural history of patients with acute MI sent home from the ED. *Am J Cardiol* 60:219–224, 1987.

Nurses' reference library: Emergencies. Springhouse, PA: Springhouse Corporation, 1985.

Perchalski DL, Pepine CJ: Patient with coronary artery spasm & the role of the critical care nurse. *Heart Lung* 16(4): 392–402, 1987.

Rea RE, Bourg PW, Parker JG, Rushing D, et al., eds: Emergency nursing core curriculum. Philadelphia: W.B. Saunders, 1987.

Riegel BJ: The role of nursing in limiting myocardial infarct size. *Heart Lung* 14(3):247–254, 1985.

Schiro AG, Curtis DG: Asymptomatic coronary disease. *Heart Lung* 17(2):144–149, 1988.

2.3 MYOCARDIAL ISCHEMIA: THE COCAINE CONNECTION

Barbara Mlynczak-Callahan, RN, MS, CCRN

Mark is a 33-year-old black male who was brought to the ED by ambulance. He is experiencing significant chest pain, 7 on a scale of 1 to 10, that began a few minutes after he injected cocaine intravenously. He states he had used a similar amount from the same supply the previous day with no unusual effects. Mark's pain is crushing in nature and radiates down his left arm and up into his left jaw. His BP is 202/110, and his pulse is 120 and irregular. PVCs were seen by the paramedic on his cardiac monitor at the rate of 6 per minute. His respirations are 26 and heaving. His skin is warm and dry, and his Glascow coma score is 15. He states he is nauseated, and he is observed to intermittently begin to retch. The paramedics have initiated an intravenous solution of D₅ in water (keeping the vein open) and oxygen by nasal prongs at 2 liters/min. Mark has been given one dose of sublingual nitroglycerin by the paramedics with no relief of symptoms. He states he has been told he has high blood pressure but does not take his medication. He drinks ½ pint of whiskey per day, smokes two packs of cigarettes per day, and is a daily user of intravenous cocaine. He states this is his first admission to the ED related to his cocaine habit. Mark's social history reveals that he is a very successful real estate agent with his own company. His wife has been contacted at her place of employment and is driving to the ED.

Triage Assessment, Acuity Level IV: chest pain sudden onset, unrelieved by nitroglycerin, continues at rest. The patient is escorted immediately to the treatment area. A subsequent 12-lead ECG done in the treatment area shows S-T depression in leads II, III and AVF indicating inferior wall myocardial ischemia.

QUESTIONS AND ANSWERS

1. **What is the physiological basis for the systemic responses being presented by Mark?**

    Cocaine is classified as a local anesthetic and sympathomimetic drug. It is an alkaloid derived from the leaves of the coca shrub which grows in Peru and other parts of South America. When a moderate amount is absorbed systemically, cocaine stimulates the CNS resulting in a fight-or-flight reaction. The pulse is stronger and more rapid, BP is elevated, respirations are faster and deeper, and the activities of the brain are increased. The patient is more talkative, is more alert mentally, and feels exhilarated. The patient's pupils are dilated, blood sugar increases, and there is peripheral vasoconstriction (1).

    In early cocaine stimulation, with moderate dosages, the effects occur from the head downward. The initial response is euphoria and restlessness. Motor activity increases with an increase in repetitive motor actions such as picking and stroking. The cardiovascular effects occur causing increased heart rate (sometimes 30 to 50% above normal), increased contractility, and vasoconstriction. An overall BP rise of 15 to 20% above normal can occur. Cocaine also stimulates the respiratory vasomotor and vomiting centers in the medulla which results in increased respiration, cold sweats, and nausea, vomiting, and vertigo. Mark's symptoms of tachycardia, PVCs, elevated BP, sweating, and vomiting may have two causes: cocaine and acute myocardial ischemia.

2. **Is there a relationship between the sympathetic nervous system effects of cocaine and the onset of Mark's myocardial ischemia?**

    Death caused by cocaine toxicity usually occurs largely because of the progressive effects on the CNS. Acute toxic effects are likely to occur if the drug is absorbed rapidly. Excessive absorption may cause headache, excitement, palpitation, fainting, and convulsions. Death usually occurs from failure of the patient to breathe or from progressive hyperthermia. The patient may progress very rapidly from advanced stimulation to significant depression of the CNS within a very brief period of time (1–4).

    Idiosyncratic cardiovascular effects of cocaine have been reported and may be related to myocardial oxygen imbalances from adrenergic stimulation of heart rate and coronary artery vasoconstriction, electrocardiographic conduction defects, and hypertension (5–7). Mark's preexisting history of hypertension may be aggravated by the use of cocaine. However, there have been other case reports of significant dysrhythmias and myocardial ischemia and infarction in young patients who have had few risk factors (8–10). Of the cases reported, when arteriograms were performed, coronary arteries were found to be normal (7–9). The mechanism of action for the primary ischemic event therefore is not clear. Effects may be related to the release of catecholamines and stimulation of platelet aggregation, sympathetic stimulation of the myocardium and increased oxygen consumption, or isolated occurrences of coronary artery thrombosis or vasospasm (10).

3. **Are the cardiovascular effects experienced by Mark related to his intravenous use? In other words, if he was taught to change how much cocaine he used and stopped injecting the drug intravenously, would he still be at great risk for another ischemic event?**

Certainly cocaine absorption is related to the dose administered and the route of administration. Cocaine can be made into a paste, liquid, powder, or crystal and taken orally, intranasally, or parenterally, or it may be smoked in cigarette form as a freebase (a purified form) (11). Street cocaine is usually combined with other substances such as amphetamines, caffeine, or lidocaine which can potentiate the effects of the drug (1, 2, 11, 12). "Crack," a very pure crystalized form of cocaine, is a new hazard to be addressed.

The effect of intravenous cocaine occurs in a matter of minutes, and its effect is dose-dependent (1, 2, 11). The effect of vasoconstriction caused by cocaine can prolong its absorption through mucous membranes (such as the nares), subcutaneous tissue, or muscle. Vasoconstriction can slow the peak effect to 30 to 60 min after use but can prolong duration of action up to 3 hr (1, 2, 11). Cocaine is rarely taken orally because minimal absorption occurs in the GI tract due to the acidity in the stomach. The cocaine user frequently progresses from intranasal to intravenous use for its rapid and intense effect.

Cocaine is primarily metabolized in the liver where it is hydrolyzed by liver enzymes and plasma pseudocholinesterases. The effects of cocaine can be more prolonged or more toxic in a patient who has liver disease (1). It is not unusual for persons like Mark to have an underlying problem with significant alcohol consumption and poor nutritional habits that may alter his liver functions. The myocardial ischemia experienced by Mark may be related to the sudden sympathetic stimulation that occurred with the injection of the cocaine. However, it is also likely that the same event would have occurred had he chosen another route of administration.

Although there are dose-related changes in peak plasma concentrations of cocaine, the timing of these levels usually remains consistent for each individual (11). In addition, as the person reaches tolerance for increasing dosages of the drug, the individual may crave more drug even though plasma concentrations remain elevated (11), hence reaching toxic levels.

4. **What nursing diagnoses are applicable to this situation?**

The patient who is experiencing acute myocardial ischemia or infarction related to cocaine use should be recognized and managed as any other patient with myocardial ischemia precipitated by other factors such as arteriosclerosis and vasospasm. However, there are additional challenges due to the direct effect of the drug on the CNS. The appropriate nursing diagnoses (13) for this patient's care are:

Diagnosis: Acute pain related to myocardial ischemia or decreased oxygen supply to the myocardium

Desired patient outcome: The patient will state that there is relief or reduction in the chest pain and does not exhibit cues of discomfort.

Diagnosis: Potential for decreased cardiac output related to life-threatening arrhythmias secondary to injury or to enhanced automaticity of the myocardium, or potential for impaired contractility secondary to myocardial muscle injury

Desired patient outcome: Patient remains in normal sinus rhythm; patient maintains a normal cardiac output as evidenced by systolic BP > 90 mm Hg and HR < 100 beats/min; patient remains oriented to person, place, and time; skin remains warm and dry; and urinary output > 30 ml/hr.

Diagnosis: Knowledge deficit related to use of cocaine, myocardial ischemia, and high blood pressure implications for life-style changes

Desired patient outcome: Patient verbalizes an understanding of the relationship between his cocaine habit and the effect on his heart; patient verbalizes an understanding of his risk factors related to his heart including diet, smoking, drug use, and management of his high blood pressure.

5. **What interventions should the nurse initiate in this situation?**

Nursing interventions for Mark are similar to those for any patient with acute myocardial ischemia. The goal is to relieve the patient's pain and anxiety and reduce cardiac work load. The nurse should assess the patient's chest pain for location and radiation, duration, intensity, quality, and chronology (precipitating factors), and other related symptoms. The patient's HR and BP should be monitored with each episode of chest pain as the sympathetic stimulation caused by the pain and by the cocaine may significantly increase both of these. However, if the patient has experienced significant myocardial muscle damage, there may be reduced cardiac output and a low BP. The sympathetic stimulation of the pain and cocaine action are also probable causes for Mark's PVCs. Mark's history of high blood pressure should be taken into serious consideration in monitoring these parameters. To relieve Mark's pain careful titration of intravenous morphine sulfate was ordered by the physician and administered by the nurse with constant reassessment of Mark's overall pain condition. Morphine is also a useful adjunct for reducing preload and the workload of the heart, thus improving cardiac output.

TIP: A low BP is not necessarily a contraindication for administering intravenous morphine to a patient. BP may be reduced related to the ongoing ischemia that is reducing myocardial contractility or the increased preload that is reducing myocardial pump efficiency.

Oxygen was ordered by the physician at 3 liters/min (usual range is 2 to 6 liters/min) for the myocardial oxygen demands. Serial 12-lead ECGs and blood samples to measure cardiac enzymes along with other routine labs are also indicated and were performed. Monitoring of cardiac output in the ED is usually through indirect measures of systolic BP and HR, skin temperature, urinary output, and the evaluation of the patient's degree of orientation and restlessness. Significant changes in these are recorded and reported to the physician for further orders.

In some cases of myocardial infarction or ischemia, interdependent nursing actions around the administration of nitroglycerin for the reduction of preload may be indicated. In the case of cocaine-induced ischemia, the therapeutic goals are to minimize nervous system stimulation and support ventilation and circulation. Intravenous propranolol (1 mg administered slowly and repeated every minute to a maximum of 6 mg) has been used to block the β-adrenergic stimulation of HR and BP (14). Because the α-adrenergic effects of vasoconstriction are left unopposed when propranolol is used, some authors recommend the use of α-adrenergic blocking agents such as phentolamine, or afterload reducing agents such as sodium nitroprusside (15). Antiarrhythmic drugs such as lidocaine may also be indicated if other measures fail to relieve or reduce the cardiac instability that may exist.

Other physiological effects of myocardial ischemia should also be considered such as fluid balance overload related to poor cardiac contractility. Although Mark did not experience this problem while in the ED, his lungs were assessed regularly by the nurse for the presence of rales and his heart sounds for S3 gallop.

Although the relationship between Mark's cocaine use and his heart attack are an important educational concern for Mark and his family, the immediate educational need in the ED should be to assist the patient and his family to acknowledge the relationship of his drug use to his current illness. Orienting Mark and his wife to important significant events of the upcoming hospitalization are indicated. His discharge teaching plan should include assisting him to recognize his risk factors for heart attack and assisting with a plan for risk factor modification including BP control. Mark will be admitted to a special telemetry unit for cardiac monitoring. He should be informed of the need for more ECGs and blood drawing to ensure his safe recovery. He should be instructed to inform his nurse immediately if his chest pain returns.

REFERENCES

1. Gay GR: Clinical management of acute and chronic cocaine poisoning. *Ann Emerg Med* 11:562, 1982.
2. Jonsson S, O'Meara M, Young JB: Acute cocaine poisoning. *Am J Med* 75:1061, 1983.
3. Nanji AA, Filipenko JD: Asystole and ventricular fibrillation associated with cocaine intoxication. *Chest* 85:132, 1984.
4. Bozart MA, Wise RA: Toxicity associated with long term intravenous heroin and cocaine self-administration in the rat. *JAMA* 254:81, 1985.
5. Coleman DL, Ross TF, Naughton JL: Myocardial ischemia and infarction related to recreational cocaine use. *East J Med* 136:444, 1982.
6. Kossowsky WA, Lyn AF: Cocaine and acute myocardial infarction: a probable connection. *Chest* 86:729, 1984.
7. Cregler LL, Mark H: Relation of acute myocardial infarction to cocaine abuse. *Am J Cardiol* 56:794, 1985.
8. Pasternak PF, Colvin SB, Baumann FG: Cocaine induced angina pectoris and acute myocardial infarction in patients younger than 40 years. *Am J Cardiol* 55:847, 1985.
9. Howard RE, Hueter DC, Davis GJ: Acute myocardial infarction following cocaine abuse in a young woman with normal coronary arteries. *JAMA* 256:95, 1985.
10. Cregler LL, Mark H: Cardiovascular dangers of cocaine abuse. *Am Heart J* 111:793, 1986.
11. Javaid JI, Fischman MW, Schuster CR, et al.: Cocaine plasma concentration in relation to physiologic and subjective effects in humans. *Science* 202:227, 1978.
12. Loveys BJ: Physiologic effects of cocaine with particular reference to the cardiovascular system. *Heart Lung* 16(2):175, 1987.
13. Swearingen PL, Sommers MS, Miller K: Manual of critical care, applying nursing diagnosis to adult critical illness. St. Louis: C. V. Mosby, 78, 1988.
14. Rappolt RT, Gay GR, and Inaba DS: Propranolol: A specific antagonist to cocaine. *Clin Toxicol* 10:265, 1977.
15. Benowitz NL, Rosenburg J, Becker CE: Cardiopulmonary catastrophes in drug overdosed patients. *Med Clin North Am* 63:267, 1979.

2.4 PRIMARY TACHYDYSRHYTHMIAS IN THE EMERGENCY DEPARTMENT

Valerie A. Barron, RN, BSN, CCRN, CEN

Rick W. is a twenty-year-old white male who walks into the triage area complaining of palpitations and dizziness. Rick tells the triage nurse, "My heart's pounding so fast. I can hear it in my ear! I feel dizzy." Rick looks anxious and pale. His breathing is slightly labored and his skin is cool and moist.

Rick is assisted with lying supine on a stretcher. His vital signs are temperature 98.2° F, pulse 180 and regular, respirations 24, and BP 90/60. Lung sounds are clear and heart sounds are normal.

Rick states he is unmarried, graduated from college 2 months ago, and is living with his parents and two siblings. He has been unable to obtain a job since graduation. Rick uses alcohol occasionally and smokes "grass" once in a while. When asked about previous health problems, Rick replies, "They told me that I had some kind of heart condition." Rick says that he has been to the hospital twice in the past for rapid heartbeats. The last episode was about 2 years ago. Rick mentions that he was instructed to return to the clinic for follow-up but never went.

Triage Assessment, Acuity Level IV: HR ≥ 150 beats/min, BP ≤ 90 systolic; dizzy.

Rick is taken immediately to the treatment area where a 12-lead ECG shows tachycardia with slightly wide ventricular complexes and no discernible P waves. A diagnosis of supraventricular tachycardia (SVT) is made. An intravenous line is established and blood samples are obtained for CBC, BUN, glucose, electrolytes, calcium, and cardiac enzymes. With physician direction and nurse support, Rick is directed in Valsalva maneuvers. These measures are unsuccessful, so the physician performs carotid sinus massage. As there is still no change in the cardiac rate or rhythm, Rick is given verapamil 5 mg intravenous push. The dose is repeated until a total dose of 15 mg of verapamil is given and there is conversion of Rick's heart rhythm to normal sinus at a rate of 76 beats/min. The 12-lead ECG taken after the change in cardiac rhythm reveals sinus rhythm with a PR interval of 0.08 sec and a QRS duration of 0.14 sec. Delta waves are noted on the upstroke of the QRS complexes. A diagnosis of Wolff-Parkinson-White syndrome is made by the ED physician.

QUESTIONS AND ANSWERS

1. What is the etiology of SVT?

SVT is a rapid heart rhythm that is initiated by an impulse above the ventricles. The term SVT is used when the precise mechanism causing the tachycardia is unable to be determined. The umbrella term, SVT, then, might include atrial or junctional tachydysrhythmias. The initial impulse originates in the atrial or junctional area and travels down the conduction system to the ventricles (antegrade conduction). The same impulse can then travel back up the conduction system (retrograde conduction). As the impulse travels retrogradely, portions of the conduction system may no longer be refractory. These nonrefractory portions of the conduction system can, therefore, be electrically stimulated by the retrograde impulse. The result is recurrent rapid depolarization of the ventricles. As this process continues in a circular fashion (down the conduction system, up the conduction system, and back down again), tachydysrhythmias are generated. This phenomenon is often termed "reentry" since the initial impulse reenters the conduction system and produces tachycardia. The impulse may reenter the conduction system through a portion of the normal conduction pathway, such as the junctional area. The original impulse might also reenter the conduction system through an abnormal extra or accessory conduction pathway. Persons with accessory cardiac conduction pathways are said to have preexcitation syndrome.

Preexcitation syndrome is a common etiology of SVT. The term preexcitation refers to early activation of the ventricles by an atrial impulse through an alternative conduction pathway. The two known types of preexcitation syndromes are Wolff-Parkinson-White (WPW) and Lown-Ganong-Levin (LGL). In both types of preexcitation, conduction bypasses the normal pathways and travels through the accessory tracts. Accessory tracts that have been identified include Kent's bundle, a direct connection between the atria and ventricles; Mahaim fibers, a connection between the junctional area and the ventricles; and James's fibers, a connection between an internodal tract and the Bundle of His (1). Conduction through these pathways is more rapid than normal, since the usual conduction system is bypassed and thus the delay at the atrioventricular (AV) junctional area does not occur. This rapid activation of the ventricles is demonstrated on the ECG by a shortened PR interval and slurring of the upstroke of the R wave or initial portion of the QRS complex. This abnormal slurring is referred to as a δ wave.

Persons with preexcitation syndrome are predisposed to developing SVT. The accessory pathways facilitate the development of reentrant tachycardias. Cardiac electrical impulses can reenter the conduction system via the accessory pathways. The result is rapid antegrade activation of the ventricles and retrograde reactivation. The cardiac impulse travels down the conduction system, back up, and then down the system again in a circular fashion. This circular movement of the cardiac stimulus is referred to as a circulating wave (2). This process is also known as "circus" movement (3).

2. **How is the diagnosis of SVT determined?**

The diagnosis of SVT is generally determined from the ECG. ECG criteria include QRS duration of less than 0.15 sec and ventricular rate of 150 to 250 beats/min. Often P waves are not discernible. If P waves can be identified, there is a regular, consistent relationship between the P waves and the QRS complexes.

The patient's clinical presentation and history may help the diagnosis. Rick's reported medical history is vague. However, preexcitation syndrome should be suspected in a young man with a history of rapid heatbeats but no history of coronary heart disease. The ECG characteristics for WPW are duration of PR interval less than 0.12 sec, the presence of δ waves, and prolongation of the QRS interval greater than 0.12 sec (4). Since the pattern of repolarization is also altered, secondary ST-T wave changes will be seen on the ECG.

TIP: Differentiating between ventricular tachycardia and supraventricular tachycardia with aberrant conduction is essential to ensure proper patient management.

The following ECG criteria support the diagnosis of ventricular tachycardia: the presence of AV dissociation; QRS duration of >0.14 sec; axis deviation (left of −30° or right of +120°); and abnormal morphology of the QRS complex such as initial taller peak ("rabbit ear") of the R wave in V1, a broad R wave, slurred or notched downslope of the S wave in V1 or V2, and a duration of more than 0.06 sec from the beginning of the QRS complex to the lowest point of the S wave (3, 5). Other criteria that favor ventricular tachycardia include presence of fusion beats, presence of compensatory pause, HR between 130 and 170 beats/min, and concordancy—ventricular complexes in the precordial leads are all negative or are all positive (6).

Most tachydysrhythmias with wide ventricular complexes represent ventricular tachycardia (2). If the ECG diagnosis of a tachydysrhythmia with wide ventricular complexes is not immediately evident, the dysrhythmia should be treated as ventricular tachycardia. Ventricular tachycardia is often incorrectly diagnosed as SVT, sometimes resulting in life-threatening conditions (7).

3. **What factors contribute to the development of SVT?**

Factors such as high caffeine intake and smoking are associated with an increased incidence of tachydysrhythmias. Overexertion and emotional stress have also been identified as possible causative agents. In addition, toxic levels of certain medications or drugs can result in tachydysrhythmias.

TIP: Solicit a comprehensive medication and drug history from the patient. If the patient is taking theophylline or antiarrhythmic medications, obtain an order for serum drug levels. If indicated, toxicology screens should also be obtained.

---

4. **What nursing diagnoses can be determined for Rick?**

The following nursing diagnoses are appropriate for Rick.

Diagnosis: Decreased cardiac output related to electrical alteration in cardiac rate and rhythm (tachycardia) as evidenced by palpitations and rapid heartbeat with hypotension

Desired patient outcome: The patient will maintain a normal sinus rhythm, BP systolic $\geq$ 90 mm Hg; HR $\leq$ 100 beats/min, urinary output $\geq$ 30 ml/hr; skin warm and dry; the patient will remain oriented to person, place, and time.

Diagnosis: Anxiety related to tachycardia and uncertainty about its effect on health status

Desired patient outcome: The patient will verbalize an understanding of current health status and activities that will help reduce anxiety. The patient will relate an increase in psychological and physiological comfort.

Diagnosis: Knowledge deficit related to heart problem as evidenced by patient's statement, " . . . some kind of heart condition"

Desired patient outcome: The patient will be able to describe type and name of heart problem, possible complications of heart problem, patient's role in management of heart problem, and when to seek medical attention for heart problem.

Diagnosis: Noncompliance related to follow-up care with known cardiac condition

Desired patient outcome: The patient will identify factors that contribute to personal noncompliance; the patient will develop strategies to reduce impediments and comply with follow-up care.

5. **What nursing interventions are appropriate in Rick's care?**

Rick's decreased cardiac output related to his dysrhythmia has the potential to become life-threatening and requires immediate intervention. The patient should be assisted to a supine position on a stretcher so that further assessment can be done and to improve venous return. If resuscitation measures become necessary, the patient will be easier to manage. Emergency equipment for resuscitation should be at the bedside. A full 12-lead ECG is recorded immediately, providing diagnostic information as well as documentation of the dysrhythmia. The patient should remain connected to the ECG machine to record various lead tracings during therapeutic interventions. Cardiac monitoring should also be initiated so that the nurse can observe the rhythm as other procedures are performed. An intravenous line should be established to provide access for medications and fluid support as needed. Since Valsalva and carotid massage maneuvers might produce severe slowing of the ventricular response, it is important to have the intravenous line in place before the maneuvers are initiated. Blood samples should be obtained, as ordered, for electrolytes, calcium, and CBC. If Rick had been on any antiarrhythmic medications or theophylline, serum drug levels would be sent to the lab. Oxygen via nasal cannula should be administered to increase oxygenation.

As the nurse performs each task, reassurance and explanations should be provided for the patient. The rationale for the treatment plan should be discussed to elicit maximal patient cooperation. The patient will need step-by-step instructions for the Valsalva maneuvers and support throughout the procedures. The patient should be told that he might feel as though his heart has "stopped" as the heart rate slows and converts from SVT to sinus rhythm.

A patient who comes to the ED with heart problems is usually very anxious. The patient needs reassurance that the health care team understands his problem and has the knowledge and skills to treat it. The nurse should give the patient a brief explanation of the nature of the problem and of the plan for treatment. In addition the nurse should explain the role of the patient in the treatment plan. As the treatment continues, the patient may feel some sense of control as he participates in his own care.

Health teaching needs include the type and correct name of the heart condition and education on the management and prevention of tachydysrhythmias. A brief description of the pathophysiology of WPW syndrome should be shared with Rick and written on paper for Rick to carry with him.

The importance of follow-up care with a cardiologist or cardiology clinic should be discussed. The nurse should explore reasons for Rick's noncompliant behavior and assist him to identify strategies to deal with these. Rick should also be instructed to avoid potential cardiac stimulants such as caffeine, smoking, alcohol, and emotional stress. Rick might be referred for job counseling if he determines that his unemployment is stressful.

6. **What other medical therapies are appropriate for the treatment of SVT? What are the particular nursing considerations associated with these therapies?**

If the patient is hemodynamically unstable, synchronized electrical cardioversion is indicated. Prior to countershock the patient should receive intravenous sedation such as with diazepam. Careful monitoring and ventilatory support should be instituted as needed.

TIP: Patients who take digoxin are very sensitive to electrical countershock and are more likely to develop ventricular tachydysrhythmias. Therefore, only small amounts of electrical energy should be used for digitalized patients. Digoxin should not be used as an antiarrhythmia medication for patients that might require countershock.

Verapamil is the usual drug of choice for the management of SVT. Verapamil is given intravenous push in increments of 5 mg doses or 0.075 mg/kg of body weight up to a total dose of 15 mg in 30 min (7). Hypotension is a common side effect experienced by patients receiving verapamil. The BP should be checked every 5 min during drug administration. Verapamil should be used very cautiously with patients who already have left ventricular failure.

Although verapamil is the usual drug of choice for SVT, several cautions should be noted. If there is any doubt about the dysrhythmia diagnosis, or if there is any suspicion that the rhythm might be ventricular tachycardia, verapamil should not be given (5). Fatalities have occurred in patients with ventricular tachycardia who were given verapamil (3).

Verapamil may shorten the refractoriness in the accessary pathways of patients with WPW (8). The shortened refractory periods can result in an acceleration of the ventricular response particularly in atrial flutter or fibrillation, and thus can produce ventricular fibrillation. Therefore, verapamil should not be given to patients with WPW and atrial fibrillation or flutter (9). In addition patients with WPW and wide QRS complexes should not be given verapamil (10).

Because Rick could not tell the nurse and physician what heart condition he had, verapamil was chosen. Fortunately, he experienced no acute side effects. For future attacks, verapamil should not be selected as first line management and Rick should be informed of this precaution. Intravenous procainamide should be used for patients with WPW and atrial fibrillation. Procainamide is also indicated for patients with wide complex tachycardias in which the origin of tachycardia is unclear.

REFERENCES

1. Lauer JH: Electrical activity of the heart: dysrhythmias. In: Cardiovascular nursing: Body-mind tapestry. St. Louis: C.V. Mosby, 1984.
2. Marriott HJL: Practical electrocardiography. Baltimore: Williams & Wilkins, 1983.
3. Conover M: Electrocardiography update. *J Cardiovasc Nurs* 2(4):45–52, 1988.
4. Zipes D: Arrhythmias. In: Comprehensive cardiac care. St. Louis: C.V. Mosby, 1983.
5. Wellens HJ: The wide QRS tachycardia. *Ann Intern Med* 104:79, 1988.
6. Karnes N: Differentiation of aberrant ventricular conduction from ventricular ectopic beats. *Crit Care Nurse* 7(4):56–67, 1987.
7. Lowenstein SR, Harken AH: A wide complex look at cardiac dysrhythmias. *J Emerg Med* 5(5):519–531, 1987.
8. American Heart Association textbook of advanced cardiac life support, Dallas, Texas, 1987.
9. Zimmerman JH, Nieminski KE: Atrial fibrillation in Wolff-Parkinson-White syndrome. *Crit Care Nurse* 7(3):84–88, 1987.
10. Erickson SL: Wolff-Parkinson-White syndrome: a review and an update. *Crit Care Nurse* 9(5):28–35, 1989.

SUGGESTED READINGS

Cook JR, Nieminski KE: Ventricular tachycardia. *Crit Care Nurse* 8(7):15–19, 1988.

Lanros NE: Assessment and intervention in emergency nursing. Norwalk, Connecticut: Appleton & Lange, 1988.

Petrie JR: Distinguishing supraventricular aberrancies from ventricular ectopy. *Focus Crit Care* 15(4):15–21, 1988.

Rea RE, Bourg PW, Parken JG, Rushing D, eds.: Emergency nursing core curriculum. Philadelphia: W.B. Saunders, 1987.

Valladares BK, Lemberg L: Wide complex tachycardia: diagnosis and treatment. *Heart Lung* 15(6):644–647, 1986.

Weller DM, Noone J: Mechanisms of arrhythmias: enhanced automaticity and reentry. *Crit Care Nurse* 9(5):42–66, 1989.

CHAPTER 3

Respiratory Health System

Overview

The respiratory health system is concerned with the movement and exchange of gases to meet cellular ventilatory needs. Assessment data in this area should include the respiratory structures, the process of breathing, and the effects of inadequate ventilation both at the level of the pulmonary vessels and on the level of cellular exchange.

Case studies selected for the respiratory health system presentation include common emergent problems. Problems patients with other respiratory complaints might have include foreign body aspiration, the pneumonias, epiglottitis, and near-drowning. Patients in this category frequently have alterations in other health systems including the neurological-cerebral and cardiovascular health systems.

CUE WORDS

AIRWAY
artificial airway
breath sounds
clearance
cough
lung aeration

BREATHING
accessory muscles
gas exchange
oxygenation
ventilation
pattern
rate and rhythm

RELATED NURSING DIAGNOSES

impaired gas exchange
ineffective airway clearance
ineffective breathing pattern
potential for suffocation
potential for aspiration

Department of Emergency Medicine Triage Protocols

Respiratory Health System

Level I	Level II	Level III	Level IV
Cough, no acute distress; cold or flulike symptoms; mild sinus congestion; resp. rate < 32, fever < 102°F	Chest pain, mild wheezing; mild resp. distress	Moderate respiratory distress; RR < 40; moderate wheezing; hemoptysis; fever > 102°F	Severe resp. distress or resp. arrest; acute wheezing; cyanosis hypoxia; RR > 40, RR < 12; color pale, dusky; using accessory muscles; severe pulmonary congestion
	Traumatic injury: blunt trauma with no resp. distress, breath sounds equal and present	Blunt trauma with moderate resp. distress; hyperventilation; uses accessory muscles	Penetrating or blunt chest trauma; hypoxia; color poor; flail chest; unequal chest expansion; crepitance; subcutaneous emphysema
	Inhalation injury: no hair singed; no SOB		Hair singed; SOB; uncontrolled cough; hemoptysis; pulmonary congestion
	Foreign body aspiration: mild cough; no SOB; foreign body sensation	Moderate SOB	Cyanosis; resp. distress; may or may not cough
	Tracheostomy: difficulty with trach management; fever < 101°F; cough with sputum production	Difficulty with trach management; SOB; thick sputum; fever > 101°F	Resp. distress; severe SOB; unable to cough secretions
			Drowning: near-drowning victim, resuscitated at scene

57

3.1 ASTHMA: AN ELDERLY PATIENT
Kathleen J. Barnett, RN, MSN, CEN

Mrs. L. is a 65-year-old black female with a previous medical history of asthma and hypertension. Mrs. L. presents to the triage nurse with a complaint of shortness of breath of approximately 2 hr duration. The triage nurse notes the presence of supraclavicular accessory muscle use and moderate dyspnea, with audible wheezes. Triage vital signs are: respirations 32, pulse 106, BP 175/110. Oral temperature is deferred because of the patient's respiratory distress and mouth breathing.

Triage Assessment, Acuity Level IV: Shortness of breath with dyspnea and tachypnea; wheezing; history of bronchial asthma.

Mrs. L. is taken immediately by wheelchair into the ED for initiation of therapy. The nurse determines that Mrs. L. is on 50 mg hydrochlorothiazide daily for hypertension; and 300 mg theophylline 3 times daily and metaproterenol (Alupent) inhaler, two inhalations 4 times daily, for bronchial asthma. Mrs. L. has no known drug allergies. Mrs. L. has wheezes generalized throughout all lung fields that are graded at +2 (0 = absent, +1 = mild, +2 = moderate, +3 = severe). Peak expiratory flow rate is measured at 90 liters/min. While initiating treatment with metaproterenol inhalant solution via nebulizer, the nurse notes that accessory muscle use is also graded at +2, and a pulsus paradoxus of 12 mm Hg is present. As ordered by the physician, blood is drawn for a theophylline level and complete blood count. Intravenous access is established simultaneously with a heparin lock. An axillary temperature of 36.8°C (98.2°F) is obtained.

QUESTIONS AND ANSWERS

1. **What nursing diagnoses are applicable to this patient?**

   Asthma can be defined as the acute, intermittent, reversible obstruction of the airways (1). Attention to airway and breathing would be foremost on the priority list for the nurse caring for an asthmatic patient. However, the perception of breathlessness and the anxiety it generates are also significant factors for the asthmatic. Close attention to knowledge deficits or short-term memory lapses in the care of the elderly is also crucial for the patient with a chronic disease such as asthma. The following list outlines pertinent nursing diagnoses for a patient such as Mrs. L.

   Diagnosis: **Ineffective breathing pattern related to bronchial obstruction or to decreased energy and fatigue**

   Desired patient outcome: The patient will exhibit a respiratory rate within normal limits, diminished or absent use of accessory muscles, and diminished or absent wheezing.

   Diagnosis: **Impaired gas exchange related to decreased alveolar ventilation secondary to bronchospasm and mucus plugging**

   Desired patient outcome: The patient's arterial blood gas results will indicate $PaCO_2 < 45$ mm Hg and $PaO_2 > 80$ mm Hg (if obtained). The patient's mucosa will be pink; skin will be warm and dry.

Diagnosis: Ineffective airway clearance related to mucus plugging and/or bronchospasm

Desired patient outcome: The patient's wheezes will be diminished or absent. The patient will be able to expectorate and/or handle secretions effectively.

Diagnosis: Altered cardiopulmonary tissue perfusion related to hypoxemia secondary to impaired gas exchange

Desired patient outcome: The patient will maintain a normal cardiac output as evidenced by systolic BP > 90 mm Hg, HR $<$ 100 beats/min, and urinary output > 30 ml/hr. The patient will remain awake, alert, and oriented; skin will remain warm and dry. The patient will not experience cardiac dysrhythmias.

Diagnosis: Anxiety related to shortness of breath or perceived breathlessness

Desired patient outcome: Patient will state that she feels less anxious and exhibits cues of diminished anxiety and restlessness.

Diagnosis: Activity intolerance related to fatigue and/or hypoxemia

Desired patient outcome: Patient is able to ambulate without dyspnea.

2. **What is asthma?**

Asthma is a disease characterized by airway obstruction brought on by smooth muscle spasm of the bronchioles and hypersecretion of mucous glands (1). Asthmatics demonstrate an increased tracheo-bronchial sensitivity to any number of factors—even laughter can induce bronchospasm (2). Infection, allergic response to inhaled antigens (animal dander, pollen, house dust, mold spores, etc.), cigarette smoking, aspirin sensitivity, exercise, cold, and stress have all been implicated as precipitating factors in asthma attacks (1).

Whatever the precipitant, it induces the bronchospasm, mucus production, and edema of the mucous membranes in the bronchioles of the asthmatic. Gas exchange is impaired, and secretions are more difficult to clear. Initially, the asthmatic hyperventilates to compensate, resulting in a slightly alkalotic pH, a $PaCO_2$ lower than normal, and a slightly lessened PaO_2 (70 to 90 mm Hg). As the attack progresses, hypoxemia worsens, while the $PaCO_2$ begins to rise due to CO_2 being trapped in the distal airways. In the asthmatic, $PaCO_2$ over 45 mm Hg and PaO_2 less than 50 mm Hg is cause for alarm, as it indicates that compensatory mechanisms have been exhausted and the patient is hypoventilating.

Generally, the smooth muscle spasm associated with asthma is reversible and is episodic in nature. However, severe, unrelenting asthma attacks that do not reverse even after 24 hr of maximum doses of traditional therapy do occur and are known as status asthmaticus.

3. **If a patient is wheezing, should it be assumed that she has asthma?**

It has been estimated that over one million ED visits and 130,000 hospital admissions per year in the United States are the result of acute asthma attacks (3, 4). It has also been estimated that 4000 deaths per year are attributable to acute asthma attacks in this country (5).

However, there are any number of conditions that may cause a person to wheeze. Bronchitis, croup, chronic obstructive pulmonary disease, acute epiglottitis, foreign body aspiration, congestive heart failure, pulmonary edema, and tracheal/laryngeal obstruction are only a few of the many causes of wheezing and should be considered in the differential diagnosis. It is helpful when a previous diagnosis of asthma has been established. However, asthma has many causes and new onset of attacks can occur throughout the life span; ED personnel should be alert to the fact that an asthmatic attack can occur in a previously undiagnosed person, and that wheezing in a known asthmatic may be caused by other disease entities. A thorough history, coupled with an accurate physical assessment, can usually discriminate between an asthma attack and other causes of wheezing.

TIP: *Lack* of wheezing is an ominous sign in a known asthmatic patient with significant respiratory distress and poor chest movement—this indicates minimal air exchange, severe airway obstruction, and/or fatigue, and requires immediate intervention[1].

---

4. **Is it safe to give adrenergic agents, such as metaproterenol, if the patient is already tachycardic? When are aminophylline or corticosteroids indicated?**

The asmatic patient frequently presents with tachycardia—a manifestation of the sympathetic response to circulating catecholamines. Tachycardia can also be a compensatory response to hypoxia or anxiety.

Adrenergic agents used for the relief of bronchospasm have varying degrees of α-, β_1-, and β_2-receptor sympathetic stimulation. β_1-receptors stimulate the heart, β_2-receptors relax bronchial smooth muscle, and α-receptors cause peripheral vasoconstriction. Epinephrine is the prototype adrenergic bronchodilating drug—it has a marked bronchodilating effect, but also marked α-receptor activity that causes elevated BP and increased pulse rate. Modified adrenergic agents that have been developed to combat asthma have greater specificity for β_2-

receptors (isoetharine, albuterol, metaproterenol, and terbutaline) and are now preferred for the treatment of bronchospasm (6). Although all sympathomimetic drugs have the potential to stimulate cardiac functioning, those delivered via nebulization and inhaled directly into the bronchial tree have several advantages: lower doses can be used, the onset of action is more rapid, and the incidence of side effects (including cardiac stimulation) is lessened (6). Since sympathomimetic drugs are recommended as initial therapy for asthma, tachycardia in and of itself is not reason to withhold adrenergic agents. If, however, the clinical picture is clouded by a low BP, altered sensorium, or significantly altered arterial blood gases, more aggressive initial therapy, including intubation, should be considered.

Theophylline compounds, including aminophylline, reduce bronchospasm by elevating cellular levels of cyclic adenosine monophosphate (cAMP). A great number of asthmatics take theophylline preparations on a regular basis either orally or parenterally. A therapeutic level of between 10 and 20 µg/ml must be attained in order to be effective. Therapeutic and toxic levels are very close for theophylline, so the nurse should be alert to signs and symptoms of theophylline toxicity: irritability, restlessness, insomnia, agitation, headache, fever, fasciculations, vomiting, and convulsions. Ventricular fibrillation and vascular collapse can also occur. Theophylline levels are altered by age, smoking, alcohol, caffeine, and a number of drugs (6, 7).

Corticosteroids are the most potent antiasthmatic drugs available, but have a high incidence of systemic adverse reactions, and are therefore used primarily in patients who have not responded sufficiently to other agents. Methylprednisolone sodium methyl succinate and hydrocortisone sodium succinate are the two parenteral forms most frequently administered, and prednisolone is usually the oral drug of choice.

Atropine has been found to be effective in treating bronchoconstriction that is vagus nerve-mediated, and may be considered when other treatments have proven unsuccessful (1). When given by nebulized inhalation, side effects of tachycardia, urinary retention, and loss of visual accommodation will be lessened.

5. **What are appropriate nursing interventions for the patient with asthma?**

Much of the treatment for the patient with asthma is dependent or interdependent on physician orders for pharmacological agents. However, the nursing care of the asthmatic includes far more than medications. Two key points should be remembered from the outset. First, an asthma attack is a potentially life-threatening event and should be treated immediately. A triage acuity level of IV is usually indicated, as demonstrated by this case. Interventions should be started rapidly, and some assessment information may need to wait until treatment is initiated and the patient is breathing more easily. Second, asthma attacks are anxiety-producing, and anxiety can lead to greater respiratory difficulty. The immediacy of interventions on the patient's behalf and the calm reassurance of the nurse can begin to allay the anxiety that can add to the patient's oxygen consumption.

Frequent assessment and monitoring are integral to care of the asthmatic. The nurse should be aware of these critical warning signs:

Previous or recurrent episodes of status asthmaticus
Previous intubation for asthma
Peak expiratory flow rate (PEFR) <100 liters/min; forced expiratory volume in 1 sec (FEV_1) <0.5 liter
Altered state of consciousness
PaO_2 <50 mm Hg; $PaCO_2$ > 45 mm Hg; central cyanosis
Pulsus paradoxus > 16 mm Hg
Little or no response to bronchodilator therapy after 1 hr
Moderate to severe dyspnea
ECG abnormalities (1, 8, 9)

Frequent monitoring of vital signs is indicated, as well as monitoring of dyspnea, wheezing, accessory muscle use, and pulsus paradoxus.

TIP: The pulsus paradoxus is the difference in millimeters of mercury between the level of pressure at which the first Korotkoff's sounds are heard during expiration and the level of pressure at which one first hears Korotkoff's sounds throughout inspiration and expiration. A difference of more than 10 mm Hg is considered significant and indicates that left ventricular function is being effected by wide fluctuations in pleural pressure between inspiratory and expiratory phases. This is usually secondary to hyperinflation in the asthmatic patient.

Arterial blood gases (ABGs) are not indicated in all asthma attacks, but may be helpful in determining treatment for a moderate attack, and are critical in a severe attack. For the patient who is elderly (such as Mrs. L.), hypoxemic, or in severe distress, a cardiac monitor should be applied to assess for rhythm disturbances. The PEFR or FEV_1 are significantly reduced in severe attacks of asthma; the PEFR measures the maximum flow of air at the outset of forced expiration, and FEV_1 measures the forced expiratory volume during the first second. One of these measurements should be frequently assessed in order to trend the extent of airway obstruction.

The patient's progress toward desired outcomes should be monitored. If little or no response is seen after several inhalation treatments, another mode of therapy should be considered. The use of a theophylline compound or steroids has been described.

Concomitantly with pharmacologic therapy, oxygen should be administered. Most asthmatics are not CO_2 retainers, and oxygen is itself a bronchodilator (1). Therefore oxygen should not be withheld, and can be given at up to 5 liters/min without concern (1, 8).

Hydration is also a key component of asthmatic therapy. Oral hydration, if tolerated, should be strongly encouraged, and intravenous hydration can be used where intravenous access is established. Keep in mind that the asthmatic may already be functioning from a fluid deficit from insensible water losses; insensible loss from the lungs will increase with hyperventilation, and diaphoresis will be greater as a result of the sympathetic response and/or fever.

TIP: The average asthmatic requires 3 to 4 liters of clear liquids per day in order to maintain adequate hydration and keep mucus secretions thin. This averages approximately 250 ml, or one 8-ounce glass, every hour while awake.

Activity should be minimized in order to decrease oxygen demand in the acutely asthmatic patient. The patient should also be placed in a sitting or high Fowler's position for maximum chest expansion and air exchange—stretchers are frequently not as appropriate for asthmatics as are chairs.

6. **How might the treatment of asthma be modified for an elderly patient?**

Asthma therapy can be more complex in an older adult such as Mrs. L. because of the changes in the body with aging. The elderly patient must be assessed for preexisting cardiac conditions and renal disease that may affect breakdown and excretion of medications, leading to toxicity.

Elderly patients have more difficulty with gastrointestinal complications of theophylline use including gastritis and reflux due to gastroesophageal incompetence. There is heightened CNS activity in the elderly contributing to insomnia, anxiety, and tremors. Steroids should be used judiciously as these may accelerate degenerative conditions that may be present (such as cataracts) or may contribute to onset of latent diabetes.

Because of short-term memory losses or reduction in analytical abilities, treatment regimen and instruction for the elderly patient should be kept simple. Complex steroid tapers should be avoided. Extra time should be spent insuring that the patient can demonstrate proper use of an inhaler.

7. **What are helpful clues to determine if hospitalization is needed?**

    If after 2 to 4 hr of therapy the patient has continued dyspnea, accessory muscle use, wheezing that has not significantly improved, pulse rate > 120 beats/min, respiratory rate > 30, pulsus paradoxus > 10 mm Hg, PEFR < 200 liters/min, FEV_1 < 1.5 liters, or abnormal ABGs, hospitalization is indicated.

    Other factors to consider to support admitting the patient to the hospital include a return visit to the ED within 48 hr of the last visit, symptoms that have persisted longer than 1 week, and history of prior episodes of asthma requiring hospitalization and intubation.

    Unlike the clinical picture of asthma in children or young adults, asthma in older individuals can be relatively resistant to treatment. This should be considered in patients like Mrs. L. when making the disposition. Mrs. L. is known by the ED staff to have frequent episodes of asthma, but is able to be managed with regular outpatient treatment. After receiving 5 hr of therapy that included nebulizations and a maintenance drip of aminophylline (her theophylline level was 9 mg/dl), she was discharged home. Because Mrs. L. lives at home with her daughter, a phone call was made to her daughter describing today's visit, treatment, and discharge plan.

8. **What discharge instructions should be given to the asthmatic patient who is successfully treated in the ED?**

    The asthmatic patient being discharged from the ED must be made aware that improvement in respiratory status to the extent that a patient can be discharged does not indicate that lung function has returned to normal. In fact, lung function may remain compromised for a week or more following an asthma attack (9). The patient may respond partially to therapy, but residual airway obstruction may put her at high risk for relapse. The patient should be told that her lung function is abnormal, and that compliance with medications, hydration, and avoidance of precipitating factors is critical to her continued improvement.

    Medication regimens should be reviewed thoroughly with the patient. If the patient is taking a theophylline preparation, she should be instructed that alcohol, smoking, and caffeine can alter the theophylline level, and therefore should be avoided. (Smoking is an airway irritant that should be avoided anyway.) Theophylline should be taken with meals to avoid gastric upset. If the patient is to take a steroid taper, the taper schedule should be clearly defined and reviewed. If inhalers are used at home, be sure the patient is instructed in their proper use. The patient should be able to return demonstrate, particularly the firing of the inhaler at midinspiration. Adequate hydration and asthma triggers for the patient should be reviewed.

REFERENCES

1. Downie RL: Obstructive airway disease. *Top Emerg Med* 8(4): 13–31, 1987.
2. Korenblat PE: Asthma: diagnosis. *Mod Med* 57:70–83, 1989.
3. Rosen P, Baker FJ, Braen GR, et al.: Emergency medicine: concepts and clinical practice. St. Louis: C.V. Mosby, 1983.
4. Tintinalli JE, Rothstein RJ, Krome RL, et al.: Emergency medicine: a comprehensive guide. New York: McGraw-Hill, 1985.
5. Eisenberg MS, Copass MK: Emergency medical therapy. Philadelphia: W.B. Saunders, 1982.
6. AMA Drug Evaluations, 5th ed. American Medical Association, Chicago, Illinois, 1983.
7. Gahart BL: Intravenous medications. St. Louis: C.V. Mosby, 1985.
8. Mowad L, Ruhle DC: Handbook of emergency nursing: the nursing process approach. East Norwalk, CT: Appleton & Lange, 1988.
9. Fischl MA, Pitchenik A, Gardner LB: An index predicting relapse and need for hospitalization in patients with acute bronchial asthma. *N Engl J Med* 305(14): 783–788, 1981.

3.2 SHORTNESS OF BREATH: SPONTANEOUS PNEUMOTHORAX

Barbara Van de Castle, RN, MSN

Nancy is a 25-year-old white female who, at the triage area of the ED, is complaining of shortness of breath and chest pain. Nancy states these symptoms began suddenly, a day and a half ago, while she was sitting down after dancing. She was fine while dancing, but the pain came on at rest. The pain is only on the left side of her chest, and the pain gets worse with each breath. On a scale of 1 to 10 the pain is a 7. Nancy is anxious and is slightly diaphoretic. Nancy states she smokes one pack of cigarettes a day and has no significant medical history. Her vital signs are respirations 34, pulse 124 and regular, BP 144/90, oral temperature 99.4° F.

Triage Assessment, Acuity Level III: sudden onset of pain and shortness of breath, moderate respiratory distress, respiratory rate 30 to 40.

An x-ray is ordered at the triage area and completed for PA and LAT chest. In the treatment area Nancy's physical assessment is completed by the treatment nurse. Nancy's breath sounds are faint, but heard bilaterally. She is obviously tachypneic. No cyanosis is present. ABG results on room air are PaO$_2$ of 67 mm Hg, PaCO$_2$ of 30 mm Hg, pH of 7.50, and a HCO$_3$ of 18, showing a respiratory alkalosis and mild hypoxia. The physician reports that the chest x-ray shows a 15% left upper pneumothorax. The diagnosis of spontaneous pneumothorax is made.

QUESTIONS AND ANSWERS

1. **What is a spontaneous pneumothorax, and how does one occur?**

Spontaneous pneumothorax is a term used to describe a sudden, unexpected collapse or partial collapse of a lung. Spontaneous pneumothorax can occur in a person who may or may not have any underlying pulmonary disease. Apparently healthy young people, usually between the ages of 20 and 40 years, often experience these events. The usual cause is rupture of either a subpleural bleb at the surface of the lung, a subclinical localized bullous disease, or an erosion through the pulmonary pleura. A bleb is a large, flaccid vesicle that when ruptured allows air to leak from the pulmonary alveoli. The causes of blebs or bullae in otherwise healthy persons is not known, but a familial predisposition has been reported. Risk factors for a spontaneous pneumothorax include emphysema and chronic obstructive pulmonary disease (COPD), blunt chest trauma, lung surgery, some forms of cancer, and smoking. Smoking increases the risk of first spontaneous pneumothorax 9-fold in females and 22-fold in males, as compared to nonsmokers. Men are 3 times as likely to develop a spontaneous pneumothorax as women. Pneumothoraces of this nature can occur during inactivity or low-activity periods and are not related to physical activity or sudden movements.

2. **What is the medical management of a spontaneous pneumothorax?**

A first-time spontaneous pneumothorax is treated conservatively if the size of the collapse is under 20% of the lung field. No chest tube needs to be placed, but the patient should be asked to cough and deep breathe at regular intervals to enhance the reexpansion of the lung. A chest x-ray should be repeated at 4 to 6 hr to observe for increasing or decreasing percentage of the lung collapse. Of course, if the signs and symptoms become worse, the frequency of the chest x-rays should increase. A baseline room air ABG should be performed and oxygen administered as needed. If the patient's signs and symptoms improve, the patient will probably be able to be discharged from the ED with close and frequent follow-up with a private physician or at a clinic. If the signs and symptoms do not improve or the chest x-ray shows an increasing percentage of pneumothorax (> 20%), the patient will be admitted to the hospital and a chest tube may be placed.

3. **What nursing care problems are present with a patient that has a spontaneous pneumothorax?**

Although medical interventions are conservative and limited at this time, the nursing care needs of this patient are significant. Nancy is at risk for further respiratory compromise and should be assessed frequently. The feeling of breathlessness that occurs with a partial pneumothorax can induce anxiety and enhance hyperventilation that could exacerbate the already present respiratory alkalosis.

Diagnosis: Impaired gas exchange related to decreased functional lung tissue with secondary tachypnea

Desired patient outcome: The patient will have a regular rate of respiration between 18 to 22 and an ABG of PaO_2 of 80 to 100 mm Hg, $PaCO_2$ of 35 to 45 mm Hg, pH of 7.35 to 7.45, and an HCO_3 of 21 to 28 mEq/L; the patient's breath sounds will be heard in both lung fields and are clear and equal.

Diagnosis: Ineffective breathing pattern related to decreased functional lung tissue, feelings of breathlessness, and anxiety resulting in tachypnea

Desired patient outcome: The patient will have a regular respiratory pattern with equal chest expansion and a rate of 18 to 22; the patient will state her breathing is easier and that her feelings of breathlessness are diminished.

Diagnosis: Pain related to altered pulmonary tissue integrity and pleural irritation

Desired patient outcome: The patient will state that the pain is absent or decreased to a tolerable level; the patient will not exhibit nonverbal cues of pain.

Diagnosis: Anxiety related to the unknown cause of her feelings of breathlessness and chest pain

Desired patient outcome: The patient will describe her feelings of anxiety and use effective coping mechanisms to manage her feelings; the patient will describe an increase in psychological and physiological comfort.

Diagnosis: Knowledge deficit related to etiology and signs and symptoms of a spontaneous pneumothorax

Desired patient outcome: The patient will describe what a pneumothorax is, how it occurs, and her risk factors; the patient will state actions that she will take to reduce her risk; the patient will state signs and symptoms of a spontaneous pneumothorax and the actions she will take if the symptoms recur.

4. **What nursing actions should be taken to support this patient?**

Nancy should receive continuous monitoring of her vital signs and respiratory function, at least every ½ to 1 hr. The nurse should assess Nancy for decreased breath sounds, increased respiratory distress, tachycardia, tachypnea, use of accessory muscles, and cyanosis. Any deterioration in the patient's condition should be reported to the physician immediately. The nurse can provide comfort measures for the patient by applying ordered oxygen and positioning the patient in an upright position to reduce the effort required to breathe. Talking with the patient at frequent intervals and perhaps having a family member stay with her should make her feel less anxious. Verbal reassurances can be made by the nurse in conjunction with various nursing activities, such as during vital-sign checks, hourly rechecks of ABGs, and auscultating breath sounds.

Concurrent documentation should be completed to obtain a total picture of the patient's progress. Current ABG results should be compared with the patient's signs of improvement. The nurse can make recommendations to the medical plan of care for the patient from her nursing assessment and knowledge of normal progression for this type of problem.

5. What information will Nancy need prior to discharge?

When Nancy is discharged from the ED, she must be aware that she could develop another spontaneous pneumothorax. If she becomes aware of recurrent signs and symptoms of a spontaneous pneumothorax, she must call her physician or go to an emergency room for a diagnostic chest x-ray and treatment. Nancy should inform her family that she has this problem and how they can help recognize the symptoms. Nancy should be told to reduce or stop her cigarette smoking. She is referred to her private doctor to help her in this process as well as to check her lung condition. Nancy can be told she will not need to limit her exercise as studies show there is no correlation between physical activity and increased incidences of spontaneous pneumothorax.

SUGGESTED READINGS

Bense L, Gunnar E, Odont D, Wiman LG: Smoking and the increased risk of contracting spontaneous pneumothorax. *Chest* 96(6):1009–1012, 1987.

Bense L, Wiman LG, Hedenstierna G: Onset of symptoms in spontaneous pneumo- thorax: correlations to physical activity. *J Resp Dis* 71:181–186, 1987.

Price SA, Wilson LM: Pathophysiology: Clinical concepts of disease processes, 3rd ed. New York: McGraw-Hill, 1986.

3.3 PULMONARY EMBOLISM
Barbara Van de Castle, RN, MSN

George, a 52-year-old black male, appears at the triage desk complaining of chest pain over his right chest that goes from front to back. The pain is described as sharp and stabbing and has lasted for 3 hr. The pain occurred suddenly while George was lying in bed this morning. The pain intensifies with deep breathing, coughing, and movement. George appears anxious, dyspneic, and has rales over his right upper and lower lobes. His respirations are 42, pulse 118 and regular, BP 150/99, temperature 101.0° F. George has a medical history of COPD and is on many medications. He has no known drug allergies. George states that his problem today does not feel like his usual exacerbation of COPD and that he has been taking his medications, including aminophylline regularly. There is no swelling or redness in George's extremities.

Triage Assessment, Acuity Level IV: Severe respiratory distress, RR > 40, accessory muscle use, and pulmonary congestion.

QUESTIONS AND ANSWERS

1. What are the likely medical diagnoses for this patient and how are they differentiated?

Since George has a history of COPD, problems such as pleural effusion, pulmonary edema, pulmonary embolism (PE), or exacerbation of his COPD should be considered. Aiso, a MI or angina should be evaluated as possible etiologies for his symptoms. A chest x-ray, 12-lead ECG, and a room air ABG will be ordered initially to aid in the medical diagnosis by the physician. George's chest x-ray showed normal changes associated with COPD. Pleural effusion, pulmonary edema, and other pathologies were not evident. A 12-lead ECG helps to identify ischemic cardiac changes as weil as changes that occur with pulmonary hypertension or pulmonary embolus. George's ECG showed changes indicating a pulmonary embolism. These changes include tall peaked P waves in leads II and III, right atrial and ventricular strain pattern, right QRS axis shift, right bundle branch block (RBBB) pattern, and ST segment and T wave changes. A room air ABG is ordered to assess the patient's oxygenation and ventilation status. Since a pulmonary embolus is suspected at this point, George's ABGs were evaluated with this etiology in mind. Unfortunately, the PaO_2 has poor predictive value in excluding a pulmonary embolus. However, a decreased $PaCO_2$ in the presence of a normal PaO_2 can increase the suspicion for a PE. George's COPD can complicate the interpretation of the ABGs. However, his reported hypoxia continues to support the potential diagnosis of PE.

TIP: ABGs can be used to evaluate oxygenation and ventilation mismatching (shunting) by evaluating the alveolar-arterial oxygen gradient [$P(A-a)O_2$]. An increased $P(A-a)O_2$ gradient is an expected consequence of acute PE.

Because George's room air ABG, chest x-ray, and ECG strongly suggest a pulmonary embolus, he was sent to nuclear radiology for a ventilation-perfusion (VQ) scan where a positive diagnosis for a PE was made. Had this test been undiagnostic, a pulmonary angiogram may have been indicated.

2. **What is a PE and who is at risk for developing one?**
   A PE occurs when material, such as a blood clot, breaks free from its attachment and circulates through the blood vessels to the right side of the heart. The clot is then lodged in the main pulmonary artery or one of its branches. Ninety per cent of pulmonary emboli come from thrombi in the lower extremities. Another source is the right side of the heart in the presence of atrial fibrillation or valvular disease. Emboli can also occur from air, vegetations, or other foreign matter. Predisposing factors to venous thrombosis and PE are venous stasis,

increased blood coagulability, use of contraceptive medication, immobilization, postoperative conditions, complications of trauma, and some malignancies.

The signs and symptoms of PE are extremely variable, depending on the size of the material or clot. These signs and symptoms range from none to sudden death caused by a massive embolus at the bifurcation of the main pulmonary artery. The classic signs of a moderately sized pulmonary embolus include unexplained dyspnea, tachypnea, tachycardia, and restlessness. Pleuritic pain, friction rub, hemoptysis, and fever are not usually present unless pulmonary infarction has occurred.

3. **What is the medical management that the nurse can anticipate for a PE?**

Treatment of PE is directed toward stabilizing the patient and preventing recurrent emboli. Prophylactic low-dose heparin is frequently ordered to begin anticoagulation. In some instances thrombolytic agents that lyse clots such as streptokinase, urokinase, or t-PA may be indicated. Thrombolytic therapy is associated with considerable risk, including untoward bleeding, and is reserved for patients with massive PEs and shock. Oxygen is given as needed to treat hypoxemia and narcotic analgesics may be given for pain relief.

Supportive measures to monitor cardiopulmonary function may be required during the acute phase of the PE, such as arterial pressure monitoring lines, cardiac monitor, Foley catheter to monitor urinary output, and a pulse oximeter to monitor capillary O_2 saturation.

4. **What nursing care problems are present for a patient with a PE?**

Even though the diagnosis of a PE can be difficult, the patient care team must act quickly to prevent more thrombi and prevent shock. George is quite anxious and is having difficulty breathing.

Diagnosis: Activity intolerance related to imbalance of oxygen supply and demand, pulmonary shunting, shortness of breath, and pain

Desired patient outcome: The patient will have a regular rate of respiration between 18 and 22; the patient will describe understanding of his allowed activity and will state his mobility limits; the patient will verbalize an understanding of the need for supplemental oxygen and medications that may increase his tolerance for activities; the patient verbalizes increased comfort and ability to perform activities.

Diagnosis: Impaired gas exchange related to bronchoconstriction and decreased alveolar ventilation and accumulation of pulmonary interstitial fluid

Desired patient outcome: The patient will have a regular rate of respiration between 18 and 22; PaO_2 and $PaCO_2$ will return to baseline for this patient. The patient will have a decrease in the amount of rales heard in the right lobes of the lung; the patient's mucous membranes will be pink.

Diagnosis: ***Pain related to pleural ischemia and irritation of lung tissue***

Desired patient outcome: The patient will state that the pain is relieved or decreased to a tolerable level; the patient will not exhibit nonverbal cues of pain.

Diagnosis: ***Anxiety related to sudden onset of chest pain and shortness of breath***

Desired patient outcome: The patient will describe his feelings of anxiety; the patient will state an understanding of his situation and demonstrate ability to focus on new knowledge and skills; the patient will describe feeling less anxious.

5. **What nursing action should be taken to support this patient?**

The nurse will continue to monitor vital signs and ABG results frequently, as ordered. Medications will be administered, and the patient will be monitored for untoward effects. The patient will need a nurse at his bedside continually, at least during the most acute stage. While there, the nurse can talk to the patient, encourage relaxation, and explain procedures and equipment. Comfort measures can be used including positioning, maintaining a comfortable room temperature, providing a damp cool cloth, and, if ordered, a few ice chips for his dry mouth. Reassurance can be a key intervention for the patient as breathlessness and pain can generate fear.

6. **What information will George need to know to prevent future pulmonary emboli?**

Prevention of venous stasis will be important for George because of his activity intolerance. A balance must be maintained so that George stays active but is not overcome with shortness of breath. Ted hose or other antithrombolytic stockings will be fitted for George even while he is in the hospital, and these will be important to maintain while at home. When George is ready to be discharged from the hospital, the nurse will need to help him identify activities that he can perform that minimize fatigue. Moderate activity combined with short rest periods will be helpful. A fluid intake up to 3000 ml/day should be encouraged.

George will need instruction on the use and complications of anticoagulant medications including the possibility of increased bleeding. George should also be instructed on the signs and symptoms of thrombophlebitis and recurrence of pulmonary emboli and actions that should be taken. The ED nursing report to the inpatient unit should include patient status and progress for each of the identified nursing diagnoses.

SUGGESTED READINGS

Bohachick P, Eldridge R: Chest pain after cardiac surgery. *Crit Care Nurse* 8(1):16–23, 1988.

Cvitanic O, Marino P: Improved use of arterial blood gas analysis in suspected pulmonary embolism. *Chest* 95:48–51, 1989.

Johnson BC, Dungca CU, Hoffmeister D, Wells SJ: Standards for critical care. St. Louis: C.V. Mosby, 1985.

Price SA, Wilson LM: Pathophysiology: Clinical concepts of disease processes. 3rd ed. New York: McGraw-Hill, 1986.

3.4 SMOKE INHALATION AND CYANIDE POISONING

Cathy Robey-Williams, RN, MS, CCRN

At 3:15 AM fire department crews were dispatched to a dwelling fire. A brick row home was found fully engulfed in flames. A second alarm was sounded. Neighbors believed that George Johnson was at home when the fire started. At 3:40 AM the rescue crew exited the home with a middle-aged black male, unconscious with agonal respirations. The paramedic crew that had been standing by began treating the patient by ventilating him with positive pressure oxygen. George had a pulse and had no apparent bleeding, so the crew quickly moved him into the ambulance to complete the secondary survey.

George was unresponsive to deep pain; his pupils were dilated and reacted sluggishly to light. His mustache and nasal hair were singed. His entire body was covered with soot, and his sputum was carbonaceous. George's skin was warm and dry, his capillary refill time delayed, color dusky, and mucous membranes gray.

The rescue officer reported that George was found in a third-floor smoke-filled bedroom with no open fire near him. It appeared that the source of the fire was the living room couch on the first floor.

As the paramedic attempted intubation, George gagged on the tube and aroused slightly. Therefore oxygen was applied at 15 liters/min via a nonrebreather mask. George's vital signs at this time were BP 160/100, pulse 110, and respirations 28. Breath sounds were heard bilaterally, with coarse rhonchi throughout all lung fields. The ECG showed that George was in a sinus tachycardia with occasional unifocal PVCs. An intravenous line was established with an 18 gauge catheter and D_5W solution infused slowly. En route to the hospital the paramedic notified the ED of George's condition, field assessment, treatment, and estimated time of arrival. The paramedic also requested and was granted an order from the ED physician for 2 mg intravenous Narcan and 25 g intravenous $D_{50}W$, to be administered en route.

Triage Assessment, Acuity Level IV: Inhalation injury, hair singed; color pale, dusky; severe pulmonary congestion.

Based on the field report, the paramedics bypassed the triage area and immediately brought George to the resuscitation area. Upon arrival George is noted to be approximately 60 years old, weighing 80 kg. George is somewhat combative, pulling at his oxygen mask and attempting to sit up on the stretcher. He is not comprehending instructions given by the resuscitation team, and he is nonverbal. George appears healthy and is ventilating spontaneously, though mildly tachypneic. George's physical exam remains the same as that reported by the paramedics, and all other systems are clear of injury.

Among the initial treatments for George in the ED are intubation, mechanical ventilation with oxygen at 100%, positive end expiratory pressure (PEEP) 5 cm, and a second intravenous line. Blood samples are drawn for routine analysis. The ABG sample as well as the venous sample drawn at the scene are both sent to the lab for carboxyhemoglobin levels for comparison. A Foley catheter is inserted.

Alupent nebulization is initiated. The team leader then uses a fiber-optic bronchoscope to visualize the damage to the lower airway. Bronchial inflammation and mucosal ulceration are noted.

George's updated ABG results are PaO$_2$ 62, PaCO$_2$ 56, and pH 7.28. The field COHb is 36% and ED COHb is 24%. Three-hundred milligrams of sodium nitrate is administered intravenously followed by 12.5 g of sodium thiosulfate intravenously.

Throughout the resuscitation George's vital signs remained stable. Hyperbaric oxygenation therapy is considered and transportation arrangements are made for a helicopter to fly George to the closest chamber, located at a naval hospital 100 miles away.

QUESTIONS AND ANSWERS

1. What is the etiology and complications of smoke inhalation?

Inhalation injury is associated with very high mortality. Smoke inhalation is the leading cause of death within the first 24 hr following exposure to fire (1).

Inhalation injury is most often present when there is a closed-space accident, with presence of heavy smoke, and the patient is unconscious. Smoke inhalation produces injury through direct heat, irritant gases, and contaminated particles that are aerosolized (2). Direct thermal damage to the lower airway is rare except in the case of victims exposed to super-heated steam. Steam has 4000 times greater heat-carrying capacity than air. Mechanisms that help protect against thermal injury include reflex laryngospasm and the efficient cooling system of the respiratory labyrinth apparatus (2, 3). Irritant gases and aerosolized contaminated particles produce the more frequent sequelae seen in the ED. Toxic gases occur from combustion (burning) and thermal degradation (melting) of synthetic materials (3). Inhalation of these toxic gases can cause damage to pulmonary tissues and alter respiratory function (3).

There are many gases that are produced in any house fire. Carbon monoxide (CO) and cyanide are highly correlated and are the most lethal. Both gases act on the systemic functions of metabolism and respiration (4).

Hydrocyanic acid is the gas form of cyanide which can be inhaled or absorbed through the skin. Hydrocyanic acid is formed through the burning of materials containing polyurethane. Polyurethane and polyvinylchloride are found in many home furnishings. Cyanide is normally present in humans in small amounts. Cigarette smoking or diet (lima beans) can increase levels slightly. Cyanide is detoxified in the liver by conversion to thiocyanate which is readily excreted by the kidneys (5). Cyanide in free form rapidly combines with ferric ion, interfering with mitochondrial oxidation. The result is a block in cellular respiration producing hypoxia at the tissue and cell level (5).

Other gases formed from the burning of polyurethane include hydrogen chloride, chlorine, and phosgene. Other irritant gases formed in the burning of other household materials such as wood, cotton, and paper are the aldehydes. Ammonia is formed by the burning of nylon. All can cause mucosal irritation and damage.

CO is the most immediate cause of death from fire and smoke (6). It has an affinity for hemoglobin 210 times stronger than oxygen (7). Inhalation of 0.1% CO in room air decreases the oxygen-carrying capacity of hemoglobin by 50%. This reduction in the oxygen saturation of hemoglobin shifts the oxyhemoglobin dissociation curve to the left. CO also binds with myoglobin thus decreasing the oxygen-carrying capability to the muscle. Loss of tissue oxygen leads to ischemia, especially dangerous to the myocardium (6).

The long-term results of CO poisoning at the cellular and tissue level are most pronounced on the CNS. CO acts on the brain to increase cerebral perfusion and increase cerebral capillary permeability, resulting in cerebral edema, increased intracranial pressure, and brain hypoxia (2, 3, 6). It is thought that the permanent neurological changes seen after CO intoxication may be due to degeneration of the brain caused by inhibition of aerobic metabolism at the cellular level, which may continue for up to 4 hr postinjury. See Table 3.4.1 for a list of CO levels and associated symptoms (8).

Smoke inhalation in general produces a range of upper and lower airway injury from minor edema to necrosis of the respiratory epithelium. Bronchospasm may occur as a direct result of airway irritation (2, 6). Inhaled particles, if small enough, gain entry into the lower airway and effect immediate changes on respiratory structures. Cilia cease functioning. Histamine, serotonin, and kallikreins are released. Surfactant activity is decreased, and mucosal edema, bronchorrhea, and sloughed mucosa cause increased airway resistance and airway obstruction (2, 4, 6).

The increase in capillary permeability that is seen after an inhalation injury lasts up to 36 hr after exposure and is caused by a release of vasoactive substances such as prostaglandins, histamine, and leukotrienes. Protein movement out of the vascular compartment changes oncotic

Table 3.4.1 Levels of COHb and associated symptoms[a]

Level of COHb (%)	Symptoms
0–10	None in healthy individuals
	Reduced exercise tolerance in patients with chronic obstructive pulmonary disease
	Decreased threshold for angina and claudication in patients with atherosclerosis
10–20	Headache, dyspnea on vigorous exertion
20–30	Throbbing headache, dyspnea on moderate exertion, difficulty with concentration, weakness
30–40	Severe headache, dizziness, nausea, vomiting, trouble in thinking, visual disturbances
40–50	Confusion, syncope on exertion
50–60	Collapse, convulsions
60–70	Coma, frequently fatal
> 70	Coma, death likely

Reprinted with permission from Martindale LG: Carbon Monoxide Poisoning. *J Emerg Nurs* 15(2):101, 1989. Originally published in *Can Med Assoc J* 133:392–396, Sept. 1, 1985.

pressure which exacerbates the fluid shift (9). To compound the problem, inhalation injury increases formation of lymph as well as increases bronchial blood flow tenfold (6). The net effect of these changes is interstitial edema, shunting, and decreased lung compliance.

The clinical course of smoke inhalation begins with acute pulmonary insufficiency which is seen immediately postburn and progresses to pulmonary edema 6 to 72 hr after injury. Bronchopneumonia develops 3 to 10 days after injury and usually coincides with expectoration of epithelial casts (6, 10).

2. **What assessment parameters can be used to determine the risk of airway compromise?**

Injury to the airway and respiratory tract can be detected within seconds of smoke exposure (11, 12). Significant smoke exposure results in immediate airway damage which is evidenced by chest tightness, hoarseness, dyspnea, tachypnea, stridor, and wheezing (1). The following signs are clear indicators for the need for aggressive airway management: facial burns, singed nasal hairs, carbonaceous sputum, and history of closed-space exposure (1, 6, 9, 13, 14). Adventitious breath sounds are not usually heard in the early phase after exposure, but are indicative of severe pulmonary damage. Even if the patient's airway is not immediately compromised, elective intubation is preferred over waiting to intubate in less than optimal conditions.

Room air blood gases often reveal mild hypoxemia with PaO_2 in the 60 to 70 range (2). Chest x-ray is of little diagnostic value in the acute phase of care (13).

Fiber-optic bronchoscopy has been identified in the literature as the best tool available to make the diagnosis of smoke inhalation.

During bronchoscopy the following are positive findings: laryngeal edema, bronchial inflammation, hemorrhage, airway necrosis, mucosal ulceration, and charring (1, 2, 6, 14, 15).

3. **What is the risk of cyanide toxicity, and how is it treated?**

Anyone exposed to enough smoke to elevate CO levels has been exposed enough to have elevated cyanide levels (4). Therefore, anyone treated for CO poisoning should routinely be treated for cyanide toxicity as well. The incidence of cyanide toxicity in smoke-inhalation victims is high, approximately 90%. If left untreated, these patients have a mortality rate of 100% (2, 4). The symptoms of cyanide toxicity include giddiness, headache, palpitations, and vomiting. These symptoms can progress to respiratory depression, unconsciousness, and seizures. Other symptoms that occur with cyanide toxicity are hypotension, hyperthermia, and diaphoresis.

Treatment of cyanide poisoning begins with the basic ABCs. Airway management, including intubation, should be performed if indicated. Humidified oxygen (O_2) at 100% should be administered along with adequate ventilatory volumes. Cellular hypoxia must be reversed (2). The antidote for cyanide poisoning is a combination of nitrite and thiosulfate. Inhalation of amyl nitrite can be achieved immediately. Once an intravenous line is established, sodium nitrite can be administered. The adult dose is 10 to 15 ml of a 3% solution. Nitrites combine with cyanide ferric ion to form methemoglobin. Sodium thiosulfate is then administered, 12.5 g in 50 ml intravenously over a 10-min period. Sodium thiosulfate removes the cyanide from the methemoglobin by conversion to thiocyanate which is metabolized by the liver.

Immediate improvement in neurological status should be noted. If symptoms persist, treatment with half the original dose should be repeated in 30 min (5).

4. **What is hyperbaric oxygen therapy, and why is it used for CO inhalation?**

Hyperbaric oxygen therapy (HBOT) is oxygen delivered while the patient is in a pressurized environment. Patients are placed in a sealed chamber which is pressurized to 2 to 3 atmospheres absolute (ATA). When the patient reaches the intended pressure, 100% oxygen is delivered either by a mask to be spontaneously inhaled or by mechanical ventilator. Treatment periods range from 35 to 90 min depending on the institutional protocol (7, 8).

Normal arterial venous O_2 content difference on room air at normal atmospheric pressure is 5 to 6% per volume with a dissolved O_2 content of plasma of 0.3% per volume. Inhalation of 100% O_2 at normal atmospheric pressure can raise the dissolved O_2 content of plasma to 2.09%

per volume, approximately meeting 30% of the tissue O_2 demands. Carboxyhemoglobin can be 50% cleared after 20 to 30 min using HBOT (16). This compares to 50% clearance on room air over 4 to 5 hr or on 100% O_2 over 45 to 80 min (7). Administering 100% O_2 at 2.5 ATA dissolves O_2 into plasma to reach a content of 5.62% per volume, enough O_2 to meet 100% of the body's needs (2, 16).

Hyperbaric oxygen therapy requires specialized equipment, including the pressure chamber and support equipment capable of withstanding increased pressure if accompanying the patient into the chamber, i.e., intravenous pumps, ventilators, monitors. This treatment also requires specialty staff trained in hyperbaric physiology, who can ensure patient safety. This staff includes engineers to manage the delivery of the desired pressure, and the nurses to prepare the patient for the treatment and to monitor the patient throughout the procedure. Centers offering this form of treatment are limited, with only 230 chambers available in the United States (8). Most centers offer monoplace chambers where patients are slid into a cylinder and the equipment and nurse remain outside (17).

The Undersea and Hyperbaric Medical Society recommends that patients like George with symptoms of intoxication should be treated with HBOT regardless of their COHb level. See Table 3.4.2 for a listing of their recommendations (8, 18).

5. **What nursing diagnoses are applicable to this situation?**
    Nursing diagnoses for the patient with smoke inhalation include:
    Diagnosis: Ineffective airway clearance related to edema of upper and lower respiratory tract
       Desired patient outcome: The patient's airway will be patent, ensured by artificial means if necessary until edema resolves.
    Diagnosis: Impaired gas exchange related to toxic gases interfering with oxygen transport and injury to mucosal lining of respiratory tract

Table 3.4.2 Undersea and Hyperbaric Medical Society recommendations for treatment of COHb poisoning[a]

1. Patients with carboxyhemoglobin levels of 40% or more should be treated with HBO even if this means transport to another facility.
2. Patients with a carboxyhemoglobin level of 25% should receive HBO treatment if a chamber is available in the *immediate vicinity*, even if symptoms are minimal.
3. Patients with signs of *serious intoxication* (alteration in mental status or neurological signs, circulatory collapse, pulmonary edema, signs of ischemia on the electrocardiogram, or severe acidosis) should receive treatment with HBO regardless of their carboxyhemoglobin levels.

Reprinted with permission from Ludwig L: The role of hyperbaric oxygen in current emergency medical care. *J Emerg Nurs* 15(3):235, 1989.

Desired patient outcome: The patient's oxygen requirements will be met as evidenced by ABGs within normal limits, PvO$_2$ 35 to 40, and O$_2$ consumption 180 to 280. The patient will be awake, alert, and oriented, and his cardiac irritability will diminish.

Diagnosis: Ineffective breathing pattern related to hypoxic effects on the CNS

Desired patient outcome: The patient will have spontaneous ventilation at a rate of 12 to 20 breaths/min. The patient's breath sounds will remain audible and clear throughout lung fields; tidal volumes will remain sufficient to maintain normal ABGs. Capillary O$_2$ saturation will be maintained above 97%.

Diagnosis: Altered cerebral tissue perfusion related to increased cerebral capillary permeability

Desired patient outcome: The patient will maintain a Glasgow coma score of 15 and a mean arterial pressure (MAP) above 80 mm Hg.

Diagnosis: Decreased cardiac output related to ischemic myocardium with decreased cardiac contractility and dysrythmias

Desired patient outcome: The patient will maintain hemodynamic stability evidenced by absence of dysrhythmias, absence of S-T elevation or depression, systolic BP greater than 100 mm Hg, brisk capillary refill, and 3+ pulses in all four extremities, and urinary output $\geq$ 30 ml/hr.

6. **What nursing interventions should the ED nurse initiate in this situation?**

Nursing interventions for George focus on maintenance of an adequate airway and supporting adequate ventilation and oxygenation until the toxic gases can be removed from body tissues. The ED nurse should immediately prepare the receiving room for a patient with an inhalation injury. The following items are checked and made ready: intubation equipment, O$_2$ placed on humidity, intubation medications drawn, intravenous solutions prepared and tubings flushed, special medications that may be required are obtained (sodium nitrate and sodium thiosulfate), and monitoring equipment and laboratory tubes and slips are prepared.

Along with ECG monitoring the nurse should provide for continuous monitoring of the patient's temperature.

TIP: Hypothermia potentiates the effects of CO (19). Hyperthermia is a complication of cyanide toxicity.

The nursing documentation that is crucial for cases like George include the prehospital report, assessment findings, treatment and procedures, and the patient's response. Ongoing documentation of monitoring parameters should include vital signs, urine output, quality of ventilation, mechanical ventilator settings, as well as a description of sputum each time the patient is suctioned. In this case, since George was being transported to another facility by helicopter, transfer information that should be documented includes facility receiving patient, physician accepting the patient, ED attending physician authorizing the transfer, updated complete assessment immediately prior to transfer, along with the name and provider level of the person in which the patient's care is transferred to. If possible, a telephone report should be given to the receiving nurse and a copy of the resuscitation chart sent with the patient.

Prior to transfer, the following procedures were done to ensure safe transport of George. George's head was elevated 45° to promote drainage from the head, neck, and trunk (2). A nasogastric tube was inserted and connected to straight drainage in order to eliminate the slight gastric distention that had developed prior to intubation. A Foley catheter was placed to monitor urine output. A baseline 12-lead ECG was done.

TIP: Elevated COHb concentrations can cause the following ECG changes secondary to myocardial ischemia: ST depression, T wave inversion, prolonged QT interval, low voltage patterns, and heart block (19).

The nurse contacted the social worker for assistance in locating and notifying the family of George's condition. The nurse also contacted Duke University's Diver Alert Network [(919) 684-8111 for emergency information and (919) 684-2948 for general information] to seek guidelines as to any other therapies or procedures that may be needed prior to transfer to the local chamber facility (8).

REFERENCES

1. Mosely S: Inhalation injury: A review of the literature. *Heart Lung* 17(1): 3–9, 1988.
2. Shirani KZ, Moylan JA, Pruitt BA: Diagnosis and treatment of inhalation injury in burn patients. In: Loke J, ed. Pathophysiology and treatment of inhalation injuries. New York: Marcel Dekker, 239–269, 1988.
3. Witten ML, Quan SF, Sobonya RE, Lemen RJ: New developments in the pathogenesis of smoke inhalation-induced pulmonary edema. *West J Med* January 148:33–36, 1988.
4. Silverman SH, Purdue GF, Hunt JL, Bost RO: Cyanide toxicity in burned patients. *J Trauma* 28(2):171–176, 1988.
5. Bayer MJ, Rumack BH, Wanke LA: Toxicologic emergencies. Bowie, Maryland: Brady Co., 1984.
6. Herndon DN, Langner F, Thompson P, et al.: Pulmonary injury in burned pa-

tients. *Surg Clin North Am* 67(1):31–43, 1987.

7. Halpern JS: Chronic occult carbon monoxide poisoning. *J Emerg Nurs* 15(2):107–111, 1989.

8. Martindale LG: Carbon monoxide poisoning: The rest of the story. *J Emerg Nurs* 15(2):101–103, 1989.

9. Mikhail JN: Acute burn care: An update. *J Emerg Nurs* 14(1):9–17, 1988.

10. Shirani KZ, Pruitt BA, Mason AD: The influence of inhalation injury and pneumonia on burn mortality. *Ann Surg* 205(1):82–87, 1987.

11. Clark WR, Nieman GF, Goyette D, Gryzboski D: Effects of crystalloid on lung fluid balance after smoke inhalation. *Ann Surg* 208(1):56–63, 1988.

12. Shimazu T, Yukioka T, Hubbard GB, et al.: A dose responsive model of smoke inhalation injury. *Ann Surg* 206(1): 89–97, 1987.

13. Haponik EF, Adelman M, Munster AM, Bleecker ER: Increased vascular pedicle width preceding burn related pulmonary edema. *Chest* 90(5): 649–659, 1986.

14. Bingham HG, Gallagher TJ, Powell MD: Early bronchoscopy as a predictor of ventilatory support for burned patients. *J Trauma* 27(11):1286–1288, 1987.

15. Hubbard GB, Shimazu T, Yukioka T, et al.: Smoke inhalation injury in sheep. *Am J Pathol* 133(3):660–663, 1988.

16. Demling RH: Burn injury. *Acute Care* 11:119–186, 1985.

17. Krings J: Hyperbaric oxygen therapy and the critically burned patient. *Nurs Manage* 18(9):80A–D, 1987.

18. Ludwig LM: The role of hyperbaric oxygen in current emergency medical care. *J Emerg Nurs* 15(3):229–237, 1989.

19. Dailey MA: Carbon monoxide poisoning. *J Emerg Nurs* 15(2):120–123, 1989.

CHAPTER 4

Gastrointestinal-Genitourinary (Elimination) and Nutrition Health Systems

Overview

The gastrointestinal (GI) and genitourinary (GU) (elimination) health system is concerned with the elimination of waste products from the body. The nutrition health system is the complement to elimination and addresses the intake of nutrients and related metabolic processes. Patients presenting to the ED frequently are experiencing nausea, vomiting, diarrhea or constipation, abdominal pain, dysuria, and other problems in elimination. Although alterations in nutritional status are not seen as frequently in the ED, anorexia, impaired swallowing, and hypo- or hyperglycemia are encountered regularly.

CUE WORDS ▬▬▬▬▬▬▬▬▬▬▬▬▬▬▬▬▬▬▬▬▬▬▬▬▬

Gastrointestinal-Genitourinary (Elimination) Health System

BOWEL	URINARY	RENAL
constipation	elimination	dialysis
diarrhea	incontinence	diuresis
elimination	hesitancy	electrolyte balance
incontinence	retention	fluid balance
ostomy	toileting	renal function
		renal stones

Nutrition Health System

INGESTION	DIGESTION	ABSORPTION AND ASSIMILATION	METABOLISM
caloric intake	abdominal distention	electrolyte balance	carbohydrate
chewing	food tolerance	fluid volume	fat
diet	gastric drainage	hydration	glucose
nourishment route	gastric enzymes	nutritional status	hormones (excluding
oral mucous	gastric motility	weight	sexual)
membranes	nausea		protein
self-care; feeding	vomiting		
swallowing			

RELATED NURSING DIAGNOSES ▬▬▬▬▬▬▬▬▬▬▬

Gastrointestinal-Genitourinary (Elimination) Health System

dysreflexia
constipation
perceived constipation
colonic constipation

diarrhea
bowel incontinence
altered patterns of urinary elimination
stress incontinence
reflex incontinence
urge incontinence
total incontinence
urinary retention
toileting self-care deficit

Nutrition Health System

altered nutrition: more than body requirements
altered nutrition: less than body requirements
altered nutrition: potential for more than body requirements
fluid volume excess
fluid volume deficit
altered oral mucous membrane
feeding self-care deficit
impaired swallowing
ineffective breast-feeding

Department of Emergency Medicine Triage Protocols

Gastrointestinal-Genitourinary (Elimination) Health System

Level I	Level II	Level III	Level IV
Diarrhea; VS normal, not orthostatic	Abdominal pain with diarrhea; VSS, no orthostasis	Abdominal pain with diarrhea; orthostasis or other clinical signs of dehydration; fever > 101°F	Severe abdominal pain with diarrhea and/or abnormal VS
Rectal itching, pain—mild; non-thrombosed hemorrhoids	Rectal bleeding, small to moderate; VS wnl; thrombosed hemorrhoids	Tarry stools or bright red blood per rectum (BRBPR); VSS, no orthostasis	Tarry stools or BRBPR with orthostasis; hypotension, tachycardia, tachypnea; rectal prolapse
Constipation		Constipation; recent abdominal surgery	Constipation with severe abdominal pain
Difficulty in starting stream of urine	Penile swelling; unable to void < 6 hr; no discomfort	Penile swelling; unable to void 6–12 hr; moderate discomfort	Inability to void for 12 or more hr
Dysuria; VS wnl; frequency, urgency	Dysuria; febrile < 102°F with or without hematuria	Dysuria; febrile > 102°F; nausea and/or vomiting with or without hematuria; no orthostasis	Gross hematuria; severe flank pain; positive orthostasis; pain suggestive of renal colic
Dialysis patient, in no acute distress, with unrelated complaint	Dialysis patient peritoneal dialysis (PD) with mild abdominal complaints; afebrile	Hemodialysis patient with abdominal complaints, febrile < 102°F; dialysis patient, problems with fistula	Hemo- or PD patient with altered mental status, seizure, syncope, cardiac chest pain, respiratory distress, bleeding, or fever > 102°F; PD patient with abdominal pain, febrile, nausea and/or vomiting

Gastrointestinal-Genitourinary (Elimination) Health System—continued

Level I	Level II	Level III	Level IV
	Abdomen distended, asymptomatic	Vomiting, febrile, dysuria, and/or urgency, with abdominal or flank pain; CVA tenderness	
		Abdomen distended, peripheral edema, no respiratory distress; diminished bowel sounds; has not moved bowels or passed flatus	Abdomen distended; respiratory distress; unable to void > 12 hr

Nutrition Health System

Level I	Level II	Level III	Level IV
Requests glucose check; asymptomatic; Chemstrip wnl	Known diabetic, c/o fatigue and weakness; Chemstrip < 250	Known diabetic, insulin-dependent; feels "funny"; VS stable, abnormal S and A, Chemstrip; history (hx) of vomiting and diarrhea	Known diabetic, insulin-dependent; change in mental status; respiratory rate decreased; Kussmaul respirations; VS abnormal
Vomiting; VS wnl; no orthostasis, no pain	Mild abdominal pain with vomiting; VSS; no orthostasis; streaks of blood in emesis	Moderate abdominal pain, guarding; vomiting and diarrhea; VS wnl but orthostatic changes or other clinical signs of dehydration; temp >101°F	Severe abdominal pain; active hematemesis; VS abnormal, hypotension; rigid, boardlike abdomen
Dysphagia; no suspicion of foreign body; no acute onset; no drooling or respiratory distress	Dysphagia; suspicion of foreign body; no respiratory distress		Dysphagia with respiratory distress

4.1 ACUTE PANCREATITIS AND THE ALCOHOLIC PATIENT

James Jay Hoelz, RN, MS, CEN

Robert is a 35-year-old white male who arrives in the ED on Sunday afternoon. Robert complains of right upper quadrant abdominal pain that he has had since awakening 4 hr ago. He states he has vomited 6 times with no relief of his pain after vomiting. He describes the pain as sharp in nature and rates it 5 on a scale of 1 to 10. He describes no hematemesis or change in bowel or urinary habits. He denies chest pain but complains of mild shortness of breath. Robert has no previous medical problems but does admit to a 20-year history of alcohol use. He admits to drinking 2 to 3 six-packs of beer every day and 1/2 to 1 pint of whiskey on the weekends. He has had pain similar to this in the past but not as severe as the present episode.

Physical examination of the patient performed by the nurse at triage reveals a thin male, somewhat disheveled in appearance. He is sitting upright, leaning forward, clutching his right upper abdomen. His speech is normal and his manner is slightly anxious but cooperative. His vital signs are temperature 100.2° F, respirations 22, sitting pulse 110, sitting BP 146/75; standing pulse 130; standing BP 130/ 60. His skin is warm and dry and his Glasgow coma score is 15. His abdomen is diffusely tender with increased tenderness to palpation in the right upper quadrant. There is an odor of alcohol on Robert's breath.

Triage Assessment, Acuity Level III: moderate to severe abdominal pain, vomiting, vital signs with 20 points orthostasis.

When the patient is brought to the treatment area, blood studies show an elevated serum amylase, an elevated WBC count, and prolonged clotting times. Robert's ABG shows a PaO_2 of 76, a $PaCO_2$ of 38, and a pH of 7.36. A diagnosis of acute pancreatitis is made by the physician.

QUESTIONS AND ANSWERS

1. What is pancreatitis, and how does it relate to Robert's symptoms?

Pancreatitis is an autodigestive disease resulting from premature activation of pancreatic enzymes. Damage that occurs within the acinar cells of the pancreas leads to an increased release and activation of pancreatic enzymes. This release of enzymes leads to local inflammation and necrosis (1). The inflammation and necrosis cause the sharp, unrelenting pain of pancreatitis. The irritation causes vomiting that does not relieve the pain (2). The pain associated with pancreatitis reaches a high intensity over a period of several hours and can persist for hours to days (3).

Pancreatic enzymes, once released, can circulate in the system at large. These enzymes can cause damage to the pleura of the lungs. Coagulopathies of the pulmonary microcirculation can occur and lead to respiratory compromise. Atelectasis, pleural effusion, and hypoxia are often complications of acute pancreatitis (1, 4).

Pancreatitis can also cause electrolyte imbalances with related patient symptomatology. As the pancreatic enzymes cause necrosis, calcium soaps are formed from fats and can lead to hypocalcemia. Circulating enzymes and necrosis can also cause damage to the β cells of the pancreas and lead to hypoglycemia from increased insulin production (5). Conversely, the serum glucose could be elevated.

2. **How is pancreatitis diagnosed? What are common causes for pancreatitis?**

In acute pancreatitis, pain is usually present and severe. It is often midepigastric, but may be difficult to localize. The pain often radiates to the back and is usually described as constant, not colicky. The patient can gain some relief of pain by leaning forward or squatting on all fours, as gravity will pull the abdominal viscera away from the inflamed pancreas. Nausea and vomiting are common symptoms. Constipation could occur, but is rare.

The patient's history review should include questions that explore the many etiologies of pancreatitis. Particularly important are a history of gallstones; use of steroids, thiazides, or oral contraceptives; endocrine disorders such as diabetes mellitus or hyperparathyroidism; or alcohol abuse (6).

Lab values that are useful in diagnosis include an elevated serum amylase, WBC count, glucose, calcium, liver function tests, and ABGs.

The serum amylase rises for the first 24 to 48 hr after onset of acute symptoms and then will begin to fall. This pattern is a useful diagnostic tool in patients who seek early medical attention (1). In some instances the serum amylase may actually be normal either due to chronic calcific pancreatitis (the pancreas can no longer produce amylase) or because of rapid clearance of the amylase by the kidney (6).

TIP: An elevated serum amylase is not exclusively diagnostic of pancreatitis. Other intra-abdominal events can also elevate the serum amylase such as perforated ulcer, perforated gallbladder, ruptured ectopic pregnancy, or diabetic ketoacidosis.

---

3. **What is the relationship between alcohol intake and pancreatitis? If Robert were to stop drinking today, would he no longer be susceptible to pancreatitis?**

Alcohol seems to increase the likelihood of damage to the acinar cells of the pancreas, thereby causing an increase in the release of destructive enzymes. Alcohol has a direct effect on inflammation and, as such, can cause necrosis. Alcohol can also directly increase pancreatic enzyme secretion (3). Together these can trigger acute pancreatitis. Robert has presented with a 20-year history of alcohol abuse.

Studies show that patients who have used alcohol to excess for 5 to 10 years or more are prone to chronic pancreatitis. It is likely that this attack of acute pancreatitis is the first manifestation of a chronic process for Robert. He could stop drinking, but he might continue to experience episodes of pancreatic pain. However, these attacks may occur less frequently than if he were to continue his present drinking pattern (7).

4. **What are the nursing diagnoses appropriate for Robert?**

Robert's problems during the ED visit center around his pain, fluid loss, and lack of knowledge about his condition. In addition, he has psychosocial problems related to his drinking that will require further analysis. For this ED visit the nurse will address the physical problems and knowledge deficit.

Diagnosis: Fluid volume deficit related to fluid loss from vomiting
<u>Desired patient outcome:</u> The patient will have no orthostasis, systolic BP $\geq$ 90 mm Hg, HR < 100 beats/min, urinary output > 30 ml/hr, good skin turgor, and moist mucous membranes; the patient will have relief of vomiting.

Diagnosis: Potential for impaired gas exchange related to coagulopathies in pulmonary microcirculation that could lead to hypoxemia
<u>Desired patient outcome:</u> The patient will have ventilation and gas exchange maintained; the patient will have clear breath sounds, respiratory rate 12 to 24, and pink mucous membranes.

Diagnosis: Pain related to inflammation and necrosis of pancreas
<u>Desired patient outcome:</u> The patient will state that there is relief or reduction of pain; the patient will not exhibit nonverbal cues of discomfort.

Diagnosis: Knowledge deficit related to the diagnosis of pancreatitis and the implications of this diagnosis to life-style changes
<u>Desired patient outcome:</u> The patient will describe the symptoms of pancreatitis and how to treat himself; the patient will describe the relationship between alcohol intake and its effect on the pancreas.

5. **What nursing interventions should the nurse initiate for Robert?**

After consultation with the physician, the nurse should provide for vigorous intravenous hydration and management of pain for the patient with acute pancreatitis. A nasogastric tube should be inserted to keep the stomach free of irritants and reduce vomiting and distension. An intravenous line should be established and fluid replacement begun. Strict intake and output measures should be taken to assess for adequate urinary output. The nurse should examine the patient's skin turgor and mucous membranes for clinical signs of fluid deficit. Hourly monitoring of the patient's vital signs should occur, and hypotension, tachycardia, and orthostatic changes should alert the nurse to inadequate hydration.

Robert's ABG results and his shortness of breath indicate a need for supplemental oxygen. The nurse should check with the physician for an order for oxygen therapy. The nurse should assess the patient's lip color and nail beds for cyanosis and any changes in mental status for early signs of hypoxemia. Breath sounds should be assessed every 2 hr. Rate and character of respirations, chest movement, presence or absence of adventitious sounds, and use of accessory muscles should be noted. Repeat ABGs should be obtained as ordered by the physician to assess the outcome of the interventions.

The insertion of the nasogastric tube may also help with pain management by reducing pancreatic stimulation and episodes of vomiting. Pain medication will also be required.

TIP: Demerol is recommended over morphine since morphine may cause spasms of the pancreatic biliary duct (8) and spasms of the sphincter of Oddi, increasing pain (1).

The nurse should assess the patient's response to pain medication. Other comfort measures may include elevating the head of the bed to a 45° angle to reduce respiratory effort, and use of relaxation techniques or massage.

Robert's teaching plan should include the disease process and answers to any questions he might have. If Robert is to be discharged from the ED, he should have an understanding of the effect alcohol has on his pancreas and his increased risk if he continues to drink. He needs to be aware of the signs and symptoms of pancreatitis and how to manage his own care at home, but he also needs to know when to return to the ED. He should be instructed in pain management techniques such as massage, relaxation, and distraction. He should also be given information on the use and side effects of any analgesics that may be prescribed. Robert should receive information on the importance of diet and nutrition versus the "empty" calories of alcohol. Finally, he should be assisted to find a primary care provider for regular follow-up.

REFERENCES

1. Sabesin SM: Countering the dangers of acute pancreatitis. *Emerg Med* 19(17): 71–96, October 15, 1987.
2. Austin J, Reber H: Answers to questions on pancreatic disease. *Hosp Med* 21(1): 141–194, January 1985.
3. Welch J: Recognizing and treating acute pancreatitis. *Hosp Med* 21(9):91–118, September 1985.
4. Barkin J, Garrido J: Acute pancreatitis and its complications. *Postgrad Med* 79(4):241–252, March 1986.
5. Cummings P, Cummings S: Abdominal emergencies, emergency nursing core

curriculum. Philadelphia: Saunders, 49–51, 1987.
6. Pousada L, Osborn HH: Emergency medicine for the housestaff officer. Baltimore: Williams & Wilkins, 144–147, 1986.

7. Greenbereger NH: Etiology and pathogenesis of chronic pancreatitis. *Hosp Pract* 20(9):83–90, September 15, 1985.
8. Adinaro D: Liver failure and pancreatitis. *Nurs Clin North Amer* 27(4):848–851, December 1987.

4.2 HYPOGLYCEMIA

Kathleen Keenan, RN, MS, CCRN

Mrs. A. is a 60-year-old white female whose family called an ambulance because she was very weak and was having trouble talking. Field interventions by the emergency medical technicians (EMT) included oxygen, consultation, and transport. Intravenous access was unobtainable. The impression of the EMTs was that Mrs. A. was experiencing a cerebral vascular accident (CVA).

On arrival in the ED, Mrs. A. is awake but unable to respond verbally. She weakly attempts to follow commands. Her pupils are equal and reactive to light, and her upper and lower extremity strengths are 1/4 bilaterally.

Mrs. A.'s past medical history, obtained from her daughter, includes type II diabetes mellitus, two MIs, and peripheral vascular disease. She was admitted to the hospital in 1986 for a femoral-popliteal bypass graft without complications. Mrs. A.'s daily medications include 40 units of NPH insulin every morning, digoxin, Lasix, and Persantine. She has no known allergies. Mrs. A.'s daughter says the signs and symptoms of weakness and slurred speech developed over several days and became most noticeable this morning. Mrs. A.'s vital signs at triage are BP 146/84, HR 122, and respiratory rate 22. Her skin is pale, diaphoretic, and cool. A finger stick blood glucose level obtained at triage is 24 mg/dl. The patient is immediately brought back to the treatment area for definitive therapy.

TIP: Any patient presenting with an altered level of consciousness should immediately have a finger stick blood glucose level checked. A patient presenting with primary psychiatric complaints may be at high risk for missed hypoglycemia. A seizure patient should also have an immediate blood glucose level performed since the seizure may be the presenting sign for hypoglycemia.

Triage Assessment, Acuity Level IV: Known diabetic, insulin-dependent with change in mental status, vital signs abnormal, blood glucose below normal.

QUESTIONS AND ANSWERS

1. **What is the pathogenesis of the signs and symptoms of hypoglycemia in this patient?**

    Mrs. A. is a type II, insulin-dependent (exogenous) diabetic. Type I insulin-dependent diabetics require insulin injections to prevent diabetic ketoacidosis (DKA). A type I diabetic, with no endogenous insulin, cannot metabolize glucose without the aid of exogenous insulin via injection. In the absence of insulin, a type I diabetic metabolizes fats which produces ketosis. A type II insulin-dependent diabetic requires insulin for control of hyperglycemia. This type of diabetic has enough endogenous insulin to be able to use glucose instead of fats as a fuel source but not enough insulin to sufficiently metabolize glucose and prevent hyperglycemia. Both type I and type II diabetic patients are at risk for hypoglycemia from their use of insulin and variations in life-style, diet, and health status.

Fasting hypoglycemia is the most common type of hypoglycemia and can result from use of such drugs as insulin, sulfonylureas, propranolol, excessive use of acetylsalicylic acid (ASA), and alcohol. Fasting hypoglycemia is also associated with hepatic failure, sepsis, and severe malnutrition, among other pathologies. Hormones involved in glucose homeostasis include growth hormone, cortisol, and adrenaline.

The signs and symptoms that occur with hypoglycemia may be divided into two categories: adrenergic and neuroglycopenic. The signs and symptoms that develop are related to the speed of the serum glucose drop, the severity of the decrease, and the duration of the event. Because cerebral cells are highly dependent on glucose metabolism, symptoms generally cluster around the neurological-cerebral effect.

Adrenergic signs and symptoms are related directly to the sympathetic nervous system's (SNS) response to an acute, rapid drop in blood glucose level. These symptoms include weakness, faintness, tremors, palpitations, sweating, hypertension, flushing, hunger, and nervousness. Neuroglycopenic symptoms occur when the fall in blood sugar is gradual or less profound. Symptoms include lethargy, personality changes, motor weakness, confusion, inability to concentrate, slurred speech, seizures, paralysis, and headache. These symptoms result from decreased cerebral oxygen uptake as the prolonged fall in blood glucose progresses.

2. **What may have precipitated Mrs. A.'s hypoglycemic event?**

Besides the etiologies already described, such as some medications, alcohol use, and some pathologies, other factors to consider when evaluating the cause of hypoglycemia for a particular patient include the type, amount, and method of administration of insulin; diet; and the eating and exercise habits of the patient. Knowing the type of insulin a patient is using helps the nurse to understand the time of peak action and duration of action.

In addition, the nurse should explore with the patient if the type of insulin being used has changed from beef or pork insulin to the newer form of insulin preparation known as Humulin. Since insulin preparations contain a number of protein impurities, a patient frequently develops antibodies to the insulin. Beef and pork insulin are known to be immunogenic, and each patient's dose of insulin is adjusted according to the individual's resistent response. The newer Humulin insulin is a more purified substance generating a reduced immunogenic response and therefore a more potent response at lower dosages. A patient whose type of insulin has been changed from a beef or pork preparation to Humulin may require an overall reduction in dose and frequency of insulin use for maximal effect and prevention of hypoglycemia.

Another concern in evaluating a patient about insulin use is to determine if the patient has changed the site of administration. If the patient switches from an area with poor absorption (poor perfusion from repeated injections) to an area of good absorption (an area with good perfusion and more rapid delivery of the drug into the circulation), the dose of insulin may actually be too high.

Patients who miss or delay meals, or eat meals lower in calories than what their insulin is intended to cover, are also at risk for hypoglycemia. The most common cause of increased insulin requirement is obesity. For the obese patient who has had insulin adjustments upward to manage this glucose load, diet adjustments should only be made with the supervision of their physician so that insulin adjustments can be made as well.

Patients who consume large amounts of alcohol have impaired glyconeogenesis in the liver which is associated with depleted glycogen stores. Compounding this effect, patients who consume a large amount of alcohol usually do not eat correctly. This combination also affects the requirement for insulin and could result in hypoglycemia.

TIP: When caring for alcoholic patients, stress the importance of eating while they are drinking to prevent hypoglycemia.

Exercise, or at least an increase from the body's normal exercise routine, can cause an increase in cardiac output and increased perfusion. Improved circulation can increase the absorption of the amount of insulin or alter its peak and duration of action and contribute to hypoglycemia.

When questioning Mrs. A. about her insulin administration and her activities over the last several days, the nurse discovered that Mrs. A. had recently begun exercising in an attempt to lose weight. Mrs. A. also admitted that she had not been following her 1800-calorie-per-day diet very well. She had been eating beyond her calorie restriction for several months, causing her to put on weight. This prompted her decision to resume her 1800-calorie diet and begin exercising this past week. She had not sought medical assistance. This change in diet and activity both contributed to Mrs. A.'s hypoglycemia, which would be considered a fasting hypoglycemia.

TIP: When patients present to the ED with complaints unrelated to their diabetes, take the opportunity in your nursing assessment to include the areas of diet, exercise, insulin administration, and glucose monitoring. Reinforce the need for medical supervision if the patient wishes to change any of these.

---

3. **What are the nursing diagnoses appropriate for Mrs. A.?**

Nursing diagnoses appropriate to the hypoglycemic patient relate primarily to the emergent problem of decreased level of consciousness. Following successful treatment, the patient's knowledge deficit should be assessed and managed. The following nursing diagnoses apply to Mrs. A.

Diagnosis: Potential for ineffective airway clearance related to decreased level of consciousness

Desired patient outcome: The patient maintains a patent airway and is free of the complications of aspiration, atelectasis, and hypoventilation as evidenced by normal respiratory rate and depth, and absence of adventitious breath sounds.

Diagnosis: Potential for injury related to decreased level of consciousness and increased potential for seizure activity

Desired patient outcome: The patient will remain free of injury as evidenced by freedom from falls and complications of seizures, and by an intact musculoskeletal system.

Diagnosis: Potential for decreased cardiac output related to current stress effect and history of MI

Desired patient outcome: The patient will remain in sinus rhythm and have an adequate cardiac output as evidenced by warm, dry skin, systolic BP $\geq$ 90 mm Hg, HR 100 beats/min, urinary output $\geq$ 30 ml/hr; and the patient will be oriented to person, place, and time.

Diagnosis: Knowledge deficit related to signs and symptoms, etiologies, and treatment of hypoglycemia

Desired patient outcome: The patient and daughter will state the causes, signs, symptoms, and self-treatment for hypoglycemia, as well as the indications for calling 911 to bring the patient to the hospital. The patient will use appropriate resources (i.e.,

Visiting Nurses Association (VNA) and private physician) for continuing follow-up and assistance in dealing with a chronic illness (i.e., proper insulin use, diet, and exercise, allowing for tight glucose control).

4. **What nursing interventions are appropriate for the patient with hypoglycemia?**

As with any physiological crisis, the ABCs have top priority. In the hypoglycemic patient, the ABCs are followed by D for dextrose. Hypoglycemia is an easily treatable problem that should be quickly diagnosed because of its potential for poor outcome. A patient with a decreased level of consciousness should be assessed for a patent airway, and cough and gag reflexes. The patient should be positioned on her side, with the head of the bed slightly elevated. Suction should be readily available. Side rails should be kept up, and the stretcher's wheels locked at all times. If the patient is restless or confused, a vest restraint is indicated to prevent injury.

Reversal of the lowered blood glucose is important to prevent further patient compromise such as seizures and cardiac arrest. Glucose may be ordered by the physician and administered intravenously or orally. The patient should be observed for the development of arrhythmias (SNS response), seizures, and coma. Because Mrs. A. has a cardiac history, she was placed on a cardiac monitor. An intravenous line was inserted. Mrs. A. was given oxygen at 4 liters/min via nasal cannula. She was administered two premixed-predosed syringes of glucose of 25 g each intravenous push. Within minutes, Mrs. A. had complete resolution of symptoms.

TIP: After treatment for hypoglycemia, the patient should be observed for signs and symptoms of recurrent hypoglycemia. If the patient is to be observed for an extended period of time, the appropriate meal tray should be ordered for the patient so that hypoglycemia will not recur.

---

5. **Why was the glucose administered intravenously rather than orally to Mrs. A.?**

The patient's level of consciousness and the severity of the SNS response need to be considered when determining which is the appropriate route for administration of glucose. If the patient's level of consciousness is depressed, as was Mrs. A.'s, or if the SNS response is extreme, the intravenous route is preferred.

Glucose is usually ordered in doses of 25 g. Twenty-five g of glucose equals 100 calories. The designation D_{50} indicates a 50% solution of glucose and water, which means that there are 50 g of glucose in 100 ml of solution or, equivalently, 25 g of glucose in 50 ml of solution. The usual dose of glucose for an average-sized adult is 25 to 125 g. If the initial dose of glucose has not reversed the symptoms, more glucose should be administered. The usual response to intravenous glucose occurs within 1 or 2 min.

Patients who are alert and able to protect their airways, and who are not exhibiting signs of marked SNS stimulation, can safely take glucose orally. Since glucose absorption occurs in the small intestine, the goal is to administer a glucose-containing drink in a form that will travel from the stomach to the small intestine as soon as possible. Sugar water or honey water is a palatable drink with a rapid GI transit time. The response to oral glucose occurs within several minutes. If the patient remains unresponsive to several administrations of glucose, consider another cause for the patient's signs and symptoms.

TIP: Prior to and during the administration of D_{50}, the nurse should aspirate on the plunger of the syringe to confirm proper line placement by blood return. If D_{50} infiltrates, it is very irritating to the tissues and could cause tissue sloughing.

---

6. **What is a reasonable period for patient observation and monitoring following reversal of a hypoglycemic episode?**

Mrs. A. was discharged from the ED within 3 hr. The reason for her hypoglycemia (exercise and diet) had been discovered, and appropriate discharge instructions and follow-up appointments had been given to the patient and family. In addition, the data collected in the ongoing nursing assessment supported the decision for discharge. The patient was able to maintain a serum glucose level between 100 and 150 mg/dl (checked at hourly intervals); the patient was alert and oriented; the patient and her family were able to describe the signs and symptoms of hypoglycemia, and they described the appropriate actions to take if hypoglycemia reoccurs.

If the cause of Mrs. A.'s hypoglycemia had not been so readily discovered, an in-depth assessment of the cause would have been indicated. If insulin or other drugs were suspect, the patient would not have been stable for discharge and may have required hospital admission for further testing and evaluation.

SUGGESTED READINGS

Alspach J, Williams S: Core curriculum for critical care nurses. Philadelphia: Saunders, 1985.

Carpenito L: Nursing diagnosis: application to clinical practice, 2nd ed. Philadelphia: Lippincott, 1987.

Dornbrand L, Hoole A, Fletcher R, Pickard C: Manual of clinical problems in adult ambulatory care. Boston: Little, Brown, 1985.

Hudak C, Lohr T, Gallo B: Critical care nursing, 4th ed. Philadelphia: Lippincott, 1985.

Kennedy P, Gerich J: Hypoglycemia: sepa-

rating fact from fiction. *Diagnosis* 10(1): 61–70, 1988.

Rosen P: Emergency medicine. St. Louis: Mosby, 1988.

Safrit H: Diagnosis: hypoglycemia. *Hosp Med* 17(2):37–44, 1981.

4.3 DIABETIC KETOACIDOSIS
Kathleen Keenan, RN, MS, CCRN

Mr. B. is a 26-year-old male who presents to the triage desk appearing acutely ill and very lethargic. The triage nursing assessment reveals sitting BP 110/88, pulse 120, and respirations 14 and deep. Mr. B.'s standing vital signs are BP 80/60, pulse 155, and respiratory rate 16.

Mr. B.'s chief complaints are nausea, vomiting, thirst, and abdominal pain. Mr. B. relates a history of type I insulin-dependent diabetes mellitus. Because the patient is lethargic, the triage nurse asks the patient about drug and alcohol use, which he denies. The triage nurse also notes a dressing on the patient's arm covering an extremely infected abrasion that the patient relates to an injury which occurred 10 days before. Additional physical assessment findings include a weak, rapid pulse; slow, deep respirations; and a dry, furrowed tongue. A finger stick blood glucose level obtained at triage is greater than 500 mg/dl. Mr. B. also states he has been having polyuria and polyphagia prior to the onset of nausea and vomiting.

Triage Assessment, Acuity Level IV: Known diabetic, insulin-dependent, with orthostatic hypotension, pulse rate > 155, blood sugar > 500 mg/dl.

Mr. B. is brought immediately to the treatment area. Initial lab results are sodium 150 mEq/liter, potassium 6.2 mEq/liter, phosphorous 0.9 mg/dl, bicarbonate 10 mEq/liter, and ABG values of $PaO_2 = 92$, $PaCO_2 = 26$, pH = 7.32.

Medical and nursing treatment focuses on the reversal of the hyperglycemia, dehydration, and electrolyte imbalance, and the treatment of infection. Mr. B. is given 2 liters of NS over the first hour of his ED stay, and then NS with 40 mEq of potassium chloride per liter at 500 ml/hr. After an initial bolus of 10 units of regular insulin intravenous push, Mr. B. is started on an insulin drip at 8 units per hr. Three hours later, Mr. B. has the following: 20 points orthostasis by pulse and BP, urine output of 20 ml/hr, lungs clear, improved alertness, serum glucose of 300 mg/dl, and positive serum ketones. Because Mr. B. remains acutely ill he is transferred to the intensive care unit.

QUESTIONS AND ANSWERS

1. What is the pathophysiology of diabetic ketoacidosis (DKA)?

Diabetic ketoacidosis is a complex pathophysiological state in which the diagnosis as well as the treatment center around reversing the hyperglycemia, ketoacidosis, and dehydration. The presence of hyperglycemia alone does not constitute DKA. Hyperglycemia combined with serum ketones signifies that fat, instead of glucose, is being metabolized resulting in metabolic acidosis. This combination of factors is essential to the diagnosis.

DKA is usually associated with a transient glucose intolerance that is the result of some stressful event. The precipitating stressor may be an infection, occasionally an MI, or noncompliance with the treatment plan. The event increases the body's production of glucagon, cortisol, and growth hormone as well as catecholamines, resulting in an overproduction and underutilization of glucose. The production of these hormones and catecholamines results in an increase of free fatty acids which produce ketones and ultimately metabolic acidosis. The glucose utilization and production, and the altered release of insulin produce severe hyperglycemia causing osmotic diuresis and dehydration to occur. Osmotic diuresis occurs through the renal tubules.

Normally the renal tubules do not "see" glucose because it is reabsorbed before it reaches the tubules. With hyperglycemia, the excess glucose exceeds the renal threshold. Some glucose is reabsorbed, but the remainder is circulated to the tubules. Because the presence of glucose makes the tubules hypertonic, large amounts of water enter the tubules to help dilute the hyperosmolar state. The glucose and water combination is then excreted in the urine. Large amounts of water and potassium are lost in this manner causing dehydration. Dehydration combined with acidosis can lead to a decreased level of consciousness for the patient, hypotension, altered respiratory pattern (Kussmaul's respirations), nausea, and vomiting.

TIP: When in doubt about the reason for a patient's decreased level of consciousness, treat as if it were caused by hypoglycemia. Administer 25 g of glucose. If the diagnosis is incorrect, the added glucose can be easily treated with regular insulin.

In addition to the acidosis and dehydration, patients with DKA often have severe electrolyte abnormalities, particularly of potassium and phosphate. When ketoacidosis occurs, potassium is shifted to the extracellular fluid as hydrogen ions move into the intracellular fluid. A large amount of this extracellular potassium is excreted through the osmotic diuresis described. Although the initial serum potassium level of a patient usually is high, there is actually a total body deficit of potassium. As treatment progresses, this deficit becomes more apparent. The use of insulin and rehydration of the patient facilitates the movement of potassium back into the cells and contributes to a lower serum potassium level. If the patient presents with hypokalemia or a normal serum potassium, there may already be a life-threatening total body potassium deficit. Phosphate, also an intracellular cation, moves in the same direction as potassium. A significant phosphate deficit may also be present.

2. **What are the signs and symptoms of DKA, and how did Mr. B.'s presentation lead the triage nurse to her decision?**

Since the diagnosis of DKA is based on the presence of hyperglycemia, ketoacidosis, and dehydration, the patient's presenting signs and symptoms relate to these three states. The patient will often describe signs of the presence of the three Ps: polyuria, polydipsia, and polyphagia. Polyuria (osmotic diuresis) leads to dehydration. Mental status changes occur from brain cell dehydration and may vary from minimal changes to coma. The slow, deep character of Kussmaul's respirations are part of the body's compensatory buffer mechanism for metabolic acidosis. These respirations can be associated with a fruity odor but should not be used as a diagnostic tool since it can be confused with the odor of alcohol and may not be present at all. The complaints of abdominal pain, nausea, and vomiting are not unusual, and are usually related to the electrolyte imbalance and acidosis. Unless a patient has an additional process going on, abdominal findings will be negative.

TIP: Documentation of baseline and ongoing abdominal assessments is important so as not to overlook acute abdominal pathology. Keeping the patient from eating or drinking will help to limit the amount of nausea, vomiting, and discomfort for the patient.

---

3. **What is the primary focus of medical treatment for the patient with DKA, and how is it managed?**

Treatment of DKA is managed through rehydration, electrolyte replacement, and insulin therapy. Dehydration and hyperglycemia can be reversed with fluid administration. Fluid administration will decrease the blood glucose level even without the administration of insulin. Fluids accomplish this by promoting glucose excretion in the urine.

NS is suggested as the initial fluid to be given. The amount and speed of the fluid replacement must be determined by the patient's status and past medical history. Most patients with severe dehydration will receive initial fluid replacement with 1 to 2 liters of NS over the first hour.

Potassium replacement is determined by the patient's initial serum potassium level. If the patient is hypokalemic, replacement should begin immediately. With normal or elevated potassium levels, replacement is usually required within the first few hours after improvement in the patient's perfusion status. Potassium phosphate may be an alternate replacement to potassium chloride thus increasing both potassium and phosphate levels simultaneously.

TIP: Potassium replacement of 10 to 15 mEq/hr or as much as 20 to 40 mEq/hr may be needed depending on the degree of deficit. The patient should be on a cardiac monitor and observed for untoward cardiac arrhythmias that occur with hypo- and hyperkalemia.

Only fast-acting regular insulin should be used to treat patients with DKA. Insulin may be administered intramuscularly, subcutaneously, by intravenous bolus, or by intravenous continuous drip. Regular insulin administered intramuscularly has a half-life of about 2 hr. This half-life generally results in a decline in blood glucose of approximately 80 to 100 mg/dl/hr. The intramuscular dose is usually 10 to 20 units per hour. If peripheral perfusion is poor in a hypotensive or dehydrated patient, the potential for poor tissue absorption should preclude the use of intramuscular insulin. There is also the risk of delayed hypoglycemia if perfusion improves and a large amount of insulin is absorbed later.

Regular insulin administered intravenously has a half-life of 20 min. Repeated intravenous bolus doses of insulin should range from 10 to 25 units per hour. Because the half-life of intravenous insulin is short, intravenous continuous drip administration is recommended. Intravenous insulin was chosen for Mr. B. because of his dehydrated state.

The insulin drip should be prepared according to hospital and pharmacy policies and procedures. In this case a drip of 100 units of regular insulin was added to 100 ml of NS to deliver 1 unit per ml, making the dosage calculation quite simple.

In administering insulin, it is important to remember that the goal of insulin therapy is not to reverse hyperglycemia, but to correct ketosis. The progressive fall in the serum glucose level should be monitored closely, along with interval monitoring of serum ketones. Insulin is still indicated to continue control of blood glucose, but it may be administered in a smaller dose or, if given by the intravenous bolus method, at longer intervals. Because Mr. B. still had ketones in his blood after 3 hr, insulin therapy was continued at 2 units per hour.

TIP: The impairment in glucose metabolism is reversed much quicker than the ketoacidosis. Even though the blood glucose may be only slightly elevated (250 mg/dl), the patient still needs insulin for the reversal of acidosis. At this glucose level the patient will require the administration of glucose in order to prevent hypoglycemia.

Mr. B.'s hand wound was suspected as the precipitating cause for his DKA. His wound was fully cultured to determine the presence of any occult infection. Wound dressings and antibiotics were started immediately. Mr. B. was given a thorough physical exam to determine if there were other causative factors such as other areas of infection. A review of his diet and use of insulin was also indicated.

4. **What are the nursing diagnoses appropriate for Mr. B.?**

Nursing care for the patient with DKA is a multifaceted problem. Attention must be paid not only to treating the presenting problem, but also to preventing complications of therapy. The following nursing diagnoses apply to Mr. B.

Diagnosis: Fluid volume deficit related to osmotic diuresis from hyperglycemia

Desired patient outcome: The patient will maintain BP and HR within normal limits, both on resting and on orthostatic assessment as evidenced by systolic BP > 90 mm Hg; HR < 100 beats/min; and urinary output > 30 ml/hr. Lab results, if available, will indicate a normal serum glucose (60 to 110 mg/dl), a normal serum osmolality (275 to 295 mOsm/liter), and a normal serum sodium (135 to 145 mEq/liter); the patient will have good skin turgor and moist mucous membranes.

Diagnosis: Altered cerebral, renal, and peripheral tissue perfusion related to dehydration

Desired patient outcome: The patient will demonstrate improved cerebral, renal, and peripheral perfusion as evidenced by an appropriate response to stimuli (awake and oriented); warm, dry skin; pink mucous membranes; urine output at least 30 ml/hr; and strong peripheral pulses.

Diagnosis: Infection related to dirty arm abrasion

Desired patient outcome: The patient will be free of infection as demonstrated by normothermia, intact nondraining skin, and clear lungs.

Diagnosis: Potential for injury related to decreased level of consciousness

Desired patient outcome: The patient will remain free of injury as evidenced by freedom from falls and an intact musculoskeletal system.

Diagnosis: Potential for ineffective airway clearance related to a decreased level of consciousness

Desired patient outcome: The patient will maintain a patent airway and be free of the complications of atelectasis, aspiration, and hypoventilation as evidenced by normal respiratory rate and depth, and absence of adventitious breath sounds.

Diagnosis: Knowledge deficit related to the signs and symptoms of DKA and its causes

Desired patient outcome: The patient and family will state the causes and prevention of DKA, including the early signs and symptoms of an elevated blood glucose level.

5. **What nursing interventions related to these nursing diagnoses are appropriate?**

Ongoing nursing assessment is critical in the care of these highly complex patients. Particular attention must be paid to identifying precipitating factors, response to fluid therapy, and the development of the potential complications of hypokalemia and hyperkalemia. Elderly diabetics are particularly prone to having an MI that may be masked by the other presenting symptomatology. A 12-lead ECG should be performed early in the treatment course and analyzed for tall, peaked T waves, and widened QRS's. The patient should be placed on a cardiac monitor and observed for arrhythmias such as PVCs indicative of hypokalemia. The patient's vital signs should be recorded at least every 15 min for the first hour and, if stable, once every hour thereafter. Urinary output should be monitored and recorded to determine that hydration and renal perfusion are adequate. The nurse should be alert to the presence of an infection, particularly of the lungs, feet, toes, and urine. The patient should be assessed for compliance with the treatment plan, and a patient teaching plan conducted, or community referrals made. For Mr. B., the nurse in the intensive care unit will continue the treatment plan and reinforce the education that was started in the ED related to infection control and signs and symptoms of DKA.

SUGGESTED READINGS

Carpenito L: Nursing diagnosis, application to clinical practice. 2nd ed. Philadelphia: Lippincott, 1987.

Foster D, McGarry J: The metabolic derangements and treatment of diabetic ketoacidosis. *N Engl J Med* 309(3):159–169, 1983.

Guyton A: Textbook of medical physiology. 7th ed. Philadelphia: Saunders, 1986.

Kappy M: Avoiding the pitfalls in managing diabetic ketoacidosis. *Emerg Med Rep* 4(15):89–94, 1983.

Lipson A: Diabetic ketoacidosis: why management is never routine. *Drug Therapy* (11):65–75, 1981.

Lueg M: Hyperglycemic dehydration: a swift but thorough approach to this subtle disorder. *Consultant* (11):91–100, 1981.

Sauve G: A primer on insulin use. *Postgrad Med* 82(3):176–179, 1987.

Swearingen P, Sommers M, Miller K: Manual of critical care, applying nursing diagnoses to adult critical illness. St. Louis: Mosby, 1988.

Tressler K: Clinical laboratory results. Englewood Cliffs: Prentice-Hall, 1982.

Whitehouse F: Diabetes mellitus: current concepts of proper management. *Hosp Med* 22(5):231–247, 1986.

4.4 RENAL STONES

Polly Thornton, RN

Mr. Thode, a 68-year-old Caucasian male, is brought to the ED in a wheelchair; he is pale, diaphoretic, and restless. He is nauseated and vomits approximately 100 ml of clear liquid immediately upon arrival. He is complaining of severe, diffuse abdominal pain.

With his family's cooperation, a triage history and assessment is completed. Mr. Thode states that he is allergic to penicillin and iodine. His BP has been normal on past routine physical examinations. At this time his BP is 154/90, pulse 96 and regular, respirations 22, and temperature 98.6° F. Mr. Thode states that he has been in considerably good health, although he had prostate surgery 8 years ago. Two days ago he experienced a sudden, sharp pain in the right flank area which resolved itself almost immediately. The pain was less severe and more localized than the pain he is experiencing this evening.

Triage Assessment, Acuity Level IV: Severe abdominal pain; pain suggestive of renal colic and/or renal stone.

The patient is taken immediately to the treatment area and prepared for a complete physical examination. The nursing assessment confirms a normal rectal temperature of 99.6° F. The patient's BP did rise to 180/90 with an increase in pain. The physical assessment of the patient confirms that he has normal bowel sounds, no abdominal distention or rigidity, and no palpable masses. Pulses (femoral, popliteal, posttibial, and dorsalis pedes) are palpable and of equal intensity bilaterally. Mr. Thode is still experiencing severe abdominal pain. The rectal examination indicates that blood is not present in the stool. The patient is put on a cardiac monitor, and intake and output measures are recorded.

Blood work is obtained and sent to the lab for CBC, electrolytes, BUN, creatinine, amylase, bilirubin, PT, and PTT. The results are reported as normal. An intravenous line of Ringer's lactate is instituted promptly with a no. 16-gauge catheter. In addition, a large bore catheter with a heparin lock attached is inserted in anticipation of a possible transfusion and as an access port for intravenous medications.

A 12-lead ECG shows an RBBB. However, there are no previous tracings available for comparison. Chest and abdominal x-rays are negative. A clean-caught urine sample is tested with a chemstrip in the ED; the test indicates there is blood in the urine. A urine specimen is sent to the lab which confirms mild RBCs, occasional WBCs, negative protein, 3+ glucose, and few bacteria. The assessment data supports the conclusion that the patient's pain is originating in the urinary system.

Approximately 1 hr after vigorous hydration, the patient, although exhausted, is suddenly almost pain-free. His color has improved and his BP has dropped to 134/ 90. Because of Mr. Thode's allergy to iodine, an intravenous pyelogram is not considered. Rather, an emergency CT scan of the abdomen is done. This procedure rules out an abdominal aortic aneurysm and confirms no gross evidence of hydronephrosis.

Mr. Thode's urologist is contacted, and arrangements are made for the patient to see him in the morning. Explicit instructions are given to the patient concerning adequate hydration, the necessity of straining all urine, the saving of any questionable stones, and the possible reoccurrence of pain. Ten 50-mg Demerol tablets are given to the patient to take home. Additional blood studies are drawn for calcium, phosphorous, and uric acid. These reports will be forwarded to his doctor.

The ED staff made a follow-up call to the patient the next afternoon. That morning, when Mr. Thode voided through the strainer provided by the ED nurses, he passed a 1.5-cm stone. He took the specimen to the urologist, who forwarded it to a laboratory for analysis. The patient was put on a low-calcium diet for several days while further testing was done. One week later the urologist also ordered a 24-hr urine collection from the patient on an outpatient basis to determine calcium and uric acid content.

QUESTIONS AND ANSWERS

1. **Which people are most susceptible to urinary calculi?**

Urinary calculi occur most often in sedentary individuals, in males rather than females (3:1), between the ages of 30 to 60, and in whites. Calculi are more likely to occur in persons living in the Southeast or the Southwest, followed by the midwest, and more so in persons living in hot, dry climates, and during the summer. Other predisposing factors include diet, recent immobilization (e.g., traction), abdominal surgery, metabolic disease, hypertension, gout, and strong family history. Patient history may include use of the following medications that may precipitate stone formation: antibiotics, allopurinol, anti-high blood pressure medications, sodium bicarbonate, phosphates, and thiazides (1, 2).

2. **What is the difference between calculi and lithiasis? Are all stones similar in composition?**

The stones themselves are called calculi; the actual stone formation is lithiasis. *Calcium oxalate* is the most common stone, occurring more frequently in men than in women. Although it is usually small, it can be trapped in the ureter. Idiopathic in nature, the stone formation is not dependent upon the urine pH. Therapeutic measures include increased hydration, reduced dietary oxalate, use of thiazide diuretics, and phosphate and calcium lactate therapy.

Struvite (magnesium ammonium phosphate) is 3 to 4 times more prevalent in women. It is usually of staghorn formation, crumbles easily, and is always associated with urinary tract infections. Struvite is the second most common type of stone. Surgical intervention is often needed to remove this stone. Antimicrobial agents and urine acidification are also considered as therapeutic measures.

Calcium phosphate stones are usually mixed, with proportions of struvite and calcium oxalate. Predisposing factors would include persons with alkaline urine and hyperparathyroidism. Treatment is the same as for calcium oxalate and struvite stones.

Uric acid stones are commonly found in men, especially Jewish males. Gout is a predisposing factor. These stones form only in acidic urine. Uric acid stones cannot be seen on x-ray without dye enhancement. Therapeutic measures include reducing the uric acid in the urine and the administration of allopurinol and sodium citrate. A diet low in caffeine, theobromine, and other purines is ordered.

Cystine stones are formed by a genetic recessive defect which causes malabsorption and excessive concentration of cystine in the GI tract and kidneys. They are formed only in acid urine, sometimes joining to form staghorn stones. Medications considered are D-penicillamine and sodium bicarbonate. A decrease in intake of milk products and a high fluid intake are advised (2, 3).

3. **Why was Mr. Thode's urinary calculus not seen either on his abdominal x-ray or on the CT scan of the abdomen?**

Stones, depending upon their composition, may be either radiopaque (cystine) or radiolucent (pure uric acid calculi). Also, a small object (in this case, a 1.5-cm stone) could be concealed easily if it were lined up with a bony prominence such as the iliac crest (4).

4. **Why did Mr. Thode experience such severe pain? Why did it suddenly go away?**

Many calculi present no symptoms for years. But when a calculus obstructs one or more calyces, the renal pelvis, or the ureter, severe back pain and/or renal colic may occur. The movement of the calculus will stimulate increased flank or costovertebral angle tenderness. The pain, which can be excruciating, can radiate across the abdomen along the ureter, down to the genitalia, and to the inner thigh. Nerve plexus and vascular density in the area increase the likelihood of diffuse, exaggerated pain. Mr. Thode was experiencing the passage of a stone through the right ureter at the time of admission, manifested as right flank pain. Complications, in the event of obstruction, include hydronephrosis and infection.

TIP: Drug addicts have mimicked these symptoms well in their quest for narcotics. A nursing assessment that includes detailed history taking and knowledge of risk factors for stone formation is very important.

5. **In an ED setting, what nursing diagnoses are applicable to this situation?**

   For the patient with a renal stone, the following six nursing diagnoses should be considered.

   Diagnosis: Pain related to the obstruction and movement of the renal calculus

   Desired patient outcome: The patient describes relief or a significant decrease in the pain experienced.

   Diagnosis: Altered pattern of urinary elimination (frequency), related to the presence of renal calculi in the ureter and the bladder

   Desired patient outcome: The patient describes relief of or a reduction in urinary frequency.

   Diagnosis: Potential for altered renal tissue perfusion, related to the obstruction of urine flow from the kidney, causing pressure in the kidney

   Desired patient outcome: The patient maintains normal renal tissue perfusion as evidenced by a systolic BP > 90 mm Hg and urinary output > 30 ml/hr; the skin remains warm and dry.

   Diagnosis: Fluid volume deficit related to nausea, vomiting, and diarrhea

   Desired patient outcome: The patient will have adequate intake (at least 3000 ml/day) and proportionate output; the patient will describe relief of nausea and vomiting.

TIP: The patient should not be excessively hydrated when having an intravenous pyelogram.

   Diagnosis: Anxiety related to concern and apprehension about pain and its cause

   Desired patient outcome: The patient describes relief from the anxiety and fear.

   Diagnosis: Knowledge deficit concerning the pathophysiological process involved concerning renal calculi

   Desired patient outcome: The patient verbalizes a working knowledge of the etiology, signs, symptoms, treatment, and prevention of his disease.

6. **What nursing interventions should the nurse initiate in this situation?**

   Nursing interventions include assessing and documenting the patient's pain—its intensity, frequency, duration, and location. Findings are reported to the attending physician. Medication is evaluated and documented. Ureteral colic is relieved by narcotics, and antispasmodics alleviate ureteral spasms.

TIP: If an intravenous pyelogram is to be done, the patient should sign the consent form prior to the administration of narcotics.

To maintain adequate hydration accurate intake and output documentation should occur. Urinary frequency is common because the bladder is stimulated by the calculus. Renal or ureteral irritation, caused by the movement of the stone, may induce hematuria. A clean-caught or catheterized urine specimen for routine urinalysis and for culture and sensitivity to rule out (or to confirm) a urinary tract infection should be obtained.

Any obstruction in the kidney or the ureter can cause a backup of urine. The patient will experience back pressure, decreased blood flow, and decreased urinary output, which will stimulate renin production. Monitor the patient's BP, since a decrease in blood flow can result in acute tubular necrosis. Renin production will raise the BP in an attempt to increase renal blood flow. Monitor lab values for elevated BUN and creatinine, and for a decreased hemoglobin and hematocrit due to overhydration.

The nurse should observe the patient's level of consciousness. Decreased movement, incoherence, and slow response to commands or to painful stimuli can indicate an accumulation of wastes and electrolytes due to inadequate filtration. These waste products and electrolytes could prove toxic to the CNS.

Renal colic causes a generalized abdominal and pelvic irritation. Nausea, vomiting, and diarrhea are frequent complaints of persons with urinary calculi. Emesis can be controlled with hygiene (mouth care) and antiemetic medications. The patient may have clear liquids and a bland diet if his tests are completed and his nausea has subsided.

Physical and emotional support must be provided for the patient. Explain the likely cause of the pain, that the stone is moving, and that, hopefully, he will be relieved of it soon. Medicate the patient on schedule or as indicated. Delaying relief of pain only intensifies it, and the patient becomes more apprehensive. When the pain has subsided, the patient can cope more easily with this illness. Assure the patient that all tests ordered are completed as rapidly as possible and that the physician is notified of the results.

The patient should be instructed in the mechanism for retrieval of the calculus. He is instructed how to use the urinary strainer and is provided with one. The nurse should emphasize the importance of retrieving any stone which might be passed, no matter how small. The nurse should advise the patient to place such findings in a dry container (if passed at home), not in alcohol, oil, or other base. Laboratory analysis will help to confirm the probable cause of the stone formation (1, 2, 4).

7. **What additional patient education and/or psychological support is required?**

The nurse should discuss with the patient and his family the importance of adequate daily fluid intake to help prevent stone formation. Six to eight liters of water may be needed. Cranberry juice will help to acidify the urine and prevent the formation of stones. If the patient is sedentary, more exercise is encouraged.

Strict adherence to a prescribed diet—usually reduced in calcium and phosphorous and low in purines—will help to reduce the reoccurrence of urinary calculi (Table 4.4.1). A high fluid intake dilutes the urine. An acid and ash diet forms slightly acid urine and helps to prevent phosphate stones. The ingestion of cranberry juice during an infection helps to form acid urine (2, 5, 6).

The patient must be urged to take appropriately prescribed drugs conscientiously.

By speaking with the patient in lay terms and with sincere concern, the nurse can help him to better understand the pathophysiology, treatment, and prevention of further stones.

There are two new procedures for removal of kidney stones that do not require major surgical intervention. The nurse should know what these are to help educate the patient and to alleviate some fear and anxiety. These are percutaneous lithotripsy (PUL) and extracorporal shock wave lithotripsy (ESWL).

Although lithotripsy would not be routine in an ED setting, it provides an innovative alternative course of treatment for the person suf-

Table 4.4.1 Foods Containing High Amounts of Purine, Calcium, and Oxalate

Purine	Calcium	Oxalate
Bacon	Beans (except green beans)	Asparagus
Chicken	Cheese	Beets
Crab	Chocolate	Cabbage
Goose	Cocoa	Celery
Herring	Dried fruits	Chocolate
Kidney	Fish	Cocoa
Liver	Foods containing flour	Instant coffee
Meat soups	Ice cream	Nuts
Mussels	Lentils	Ovaltine
Salmon	Milk	Parsley
Sardines	Nuts	Runner beans
Sweetbreads	Ovaltine	Rhubarb
Veal	Yogurt	Spinach
Venison		Tea
		Tomatoes

fering from hydronephrosis and/or severe infection due to the presence of renal calculi. In the past, the patient frequently had to withstand the trauma of major surgery and spend several weeks recuperating at home.

As opposed to surgery, PUL offers an easier, less traumatic means of removal by pulverizing the stone with ultrasound.

The PUL procedure (Fig. 4.4.1) involves the insertion of a nephroscope into the portion of the kidney where the stone is lodged. Initial attempts are made to grasp and break the stone without ultrasound. If these are unsuccessful, a hollow probe is used which sends out high-frequency sound waves that shatter the stone. With constant irrigation and suctioning the stone is removed.

PUL is not a painless procedure. The patient experiences more colicky, severe pain than that experienced after conventional surgery.

ESWL is entirely noninvasive. There is no surgery involved. The patient is immersed in water and the kidney stones are shattered by shock waves which are produced by an underwater electrode. The equipment for this procedure costs more than a million dollars, whereas the equipment for PUL therapy costs about $15,000. Both procedures, now being done in major university settings, are being brought into local communities. However, it is quite obvious that PUL therapy will be more popular because of its lower cost (3, 7).

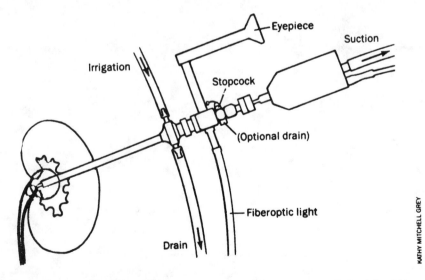

Figure 4.4.1. Basic mechanisms of a lithotriptor. (From Harwood C: Pulverizing kidney stones: What you should know about lithotripsy. *RN* July 1985:35. Copyright © 1985, Medical Economics Company Inc., Oradell, NJ. Reprinted by permission.)

REFERENCES

1. Doenges ME, Jeffries MF, Moorhouse MF: Urology: Urolithiasis. Nursing Care Plans. 11th printing. Philadelphia: Davis, 426–432, 1988.
2. Barhydt SJ, Bradley JW: Medical-surgical nursing: assessment and management of clinical problems. New York: McGraw-Hill, 1163–1169, 1987.
3. Harwood C: Pulverizing kidney stones: What you should know about lithotripsy. *RN* 32–37, July 1985.
4. Orland M, Saltman R, eds. Nephrolithiasis. Manual of medical therapeutics, 25th ed. St. Louis, Washington University, School of Medicine, 191–192, 1986.
5. Skidmore-Roth L, Jaffe M: Renal calculi/urolithiasis. Medical-surgical nursing care plans. Norwalk, CT: Appleton-Century-Crofts, 293–296, 1986.
6. Zeman F: Renal calculi. Clinical nutrition and dietetics. Lexington, MA: Collamore Press, 262–264, 1983.
7. LaCorte A, Powley M: Percutaneous lithotripsy for urinary calculi. *Amer J Nurs* 772, July 1985.

CHAPTER 5
Structural Health System

Overview

The structural health system relates to an individual's protective, physiological defense mechanisms (skin, bone, muscles, immune system). Alterations in structural integrity can give rise to potential alterations in other health parameters such as the cardiovascular and respiratory systems. Usual assessments in this area include skin breaks, joint and bone pain, strains, and fractures. Structural integrity also includes the immune system with potential for poor patient outcome when breakdown in the immune system occurs. Allergic reactions are one example of patient conditions addressed in this health system. The patient with acquired immune deficiency syndrome (AIDS) also has an alteration in the immune system that may be the etiology for the patient's primary presenting complaint. Patients with AIDS are evaluated according to their presenting complaint and triaged according to the significance of the problem in that health system. For example the patient with pneumocystis who presents with acute shortness of breath (SOB) would be triaged and managed according to the degree of dyspnea and compromise in the respiratory health system.

Case studies for this section were selected to address the wide range of presentations seen in the ED including alterations in skin and tissue integrity, breakdown of thermoregulation, and response of the immune system to an antigen.

CUE WORDS

IMMUNE	MUSCULOSKELETAL	SKIN AND TISSUE
antigen-antibody	bones	entry-exit site
body temperature	exercise	incision
immunosuppression	gait	injury
infection	mobility	tumor
inflammation	muscles	wound
leukocytes		hygiene

RELATED NURSING DIAGNOSES

potential for infection
potential for altered body temperature
hypothermia
hyperthermia
ineffective thermoregulation
potential for trauma
disuse syndrome
potential for poisoning

impaired tissue integrity
impaired skin integrity
potential impaired skin integrity
impaired physical mobility
potential activity intolerance
bathing and hygiene self-care deficit
dressing and grooming self-care deficit

Department of Emergency Medicine Triage Protocols

Structural Health System

Level I	Level II	Level III	Level IV
Distal extremity injury, no gross deformity; circulation (C), sensation (S), mobility (M) intact; pain with motion, weight-bearing; client does not appear ill	Distal extremity injury, no gross deformity; C,S,M intact; with or without edema or ecchymosis; pain, but client does not appear ill	Distal extremity injury, grossly deformed, moderate pain; C, S, M intact; client appears ill	Distal extremity injury, gross deformity; pain is severe; C, S, M deficit; client appears shocky
Laceration, superficial; C, S, M intact distal to injury; hemostasis has been or can be achieved by direct pressure; no other symptoms (sx); minor puncture wounds	Laceration; C, S, M intact distal to injury; hemostasis has been or can be achieved by direct pressure		Laceration, deep or extensive, arterial or uncontrollable venous bleeding; C, S, M deficit distal to injury; wound grossly contaminated; significant crush or avulsion injuries; trunk lacerations associated with evisceration; partial or complete amputation; open fracture; any laceration which is self-inflicted; puncture with foreign body
Minor bites, small punctures or scratches; localized insect bites		Bite, minor tear or lacerations of face; insect bites, localized allergic response; hx snake or spider bite; no distress but wound obvious	Bite, multiple lacerations, severe injury; insect bites—systemic allergic response or respiratory distress; history (hx) snake or spider bite; client appears ill; complains of pain

111

Localized wound infection; localized cellulitis; patient appears well	Cellulitis or wound infection; client febrile; appears ill	Cellulitis or infection of face or periorbital area
Thermal injury; mild discomfort; first-degree burns or sunburn comprising less than 10% of BSA	Thermal injury; moderate discomfort; first-degree burns greater than 10% but less than 25% of BSA	Any second- and third-degree burns; first-degree burns comprising greater than 25% of BSA; electrical burns; chemical burns
Complains of feeling overheated after activity; temperature less than 102°F; VSS; no hx of metabolic disease; age less than 50 years of age; cramping of most-worked muscles after exercising; weakness, headache, nausea, oriented x3	Heat exhaustion; core temperature greater than 102°F; recent history of exercise; oriented x3; headache; anorexia; thirst; vomiting; may have orthostatic changes	Heat stroke; core temperature greater than 104°F; altered mental status; no perspiration present; hot, dry skin; tachypnea, tachycardia, hypotension
	Mild hypothermia; temperature 32–35°C (90–95°F)	Severe hypothermia; temperature 30°C (<90°F)
Allergic reaction—mild itching, diffuse reaction, mild distress	Same Sx as II with hx of previous reaction to similar substance noted	Respiratory distress, ingestion of known allergen
Severe local reaction; bee sting greater than 24 hr old; no other associated symptoms	Severe local reaction with sting less than 24 hr old or with history of previous systemic allergic reaction	Respiratory distress after sting; generalized hives; gross swelling of face
Bee sting; mild local reaction; no hx of previous allergic reactions		

Fever less than 102°F	Fever more than 102°F, but less than 104°F; hx of flulike symptoms			Fever more than or equal to 105°F
Partial laceration of tongue or cheek bite; minimal bleeding or injury				Puncture wound of soft palate; amputated tongue or tip of tongue; large laceration to cheek; hoarseness with hx of trauma to larynx
Multiple minor mouth sores; no history of immunosuppression	Multiple minor mouth sores; unable to take fluid for 12 hr with no orthostasis	Same Sx as II with clinical signs of dehydration		
Sore throat, swollen glands, laryngitis; temperature < 102°F; can swallow liquids	Sore throat, swollen glands, laryngitis; temperature > 102°F; can swallow liquids	Same Sx as II with inability to swallow liquids and orthostasis		Sore throat with stridor and drooling; difficulty breathing; bleeding post T and A
Mild toothache	Toothache, fever, swelling; moderate pain	Tooth knocked out; facial or jaw pain, bleeding		Multiple teeth knocked out; mouth injury with bleeding
Bleeding gums; not on anticoagulants	Moderate bleeding gums; not orthostatic; not on anticoagulants	Significantly bleeding gums; on anticoagulants		
Requests HIV testing: asymptomatic				

5.1 SOFT TISSUE ABSCESSES:
THE INTRAVENOUS DRUG USER
Susan C. Roberson, RN, MSN, CRNP

Tanya is a 23-year-old black female who presents alone to the ED with a chief complaint of a "boil" in her right arm for 2 days. She complains of severe pain, feeling hot and cold, sweating at night, and malaise. Whispering, she admits to daily intravenous use of cocaine and heroin over the past 6 months. Tanya steals drugs from her husband, who is a dealer, but is not himself a user. She states her husband is unaware of her addiction and that she is very afraid for him to find out since she believes he would then end their relationship. Tanya reports that she is not close to her family, has few friends, and no one else she can turn to for support. She waited 2 days before coming to the ED fearing that her husband would find out about her drug-related illness. She states she injected her last cocaine dose 4 days ago in the area where the boil now is. She drinks a quart of beer about 4 times a week and smokes half a pack of cigarettes a day. She has no regular medical provider. She has no known drug allergies and no other medical illnesses. She does not remember her last tetanus toxoid immunization. This is the first negative medical sequela of her drug use.

On physical exam Tanya appears uncomfortable and anxious. She is intermittently tearful. Her vital signs are temperature 100.1° F, respirations 20, pulse 100, and BP 136/88. She reluctantly rolls up the left sleeve of her blouse to reveal her boil. At her left antecubital space is a 3-cm-diameter fluctuant abscess surrounded by 3 cm of induration, erythema, and heat. Her epitrochlear lymph node is enlarged and tender. Auxiliary nodes are not palpable or tender. There is pain with flexion of her elbow. She retains normal sensation and motor function of her hand and has normal radial and ulnar pulses.

Triage Assessment, Acuity Level III: Cellulitis and/or wound infection, patient febrile, appears ill.

Tanya was taken to the ED treatment area, and an evaluation was performed by a nurse practitioner. After her medical and social history were obtained, a physical exam was performed. Initial laboratory studies were completed, a problem list was compiled, and interventions were planned and implemented.

QUESTIONS AND ANSWERS

1. **What is an abscess, and what are the physiological processes involved in the course of its progression?**

   With the current epidemic of parenteral narcotic abuse, the urban ED nurse is frequently confronted with the overwhelming health care needs of the addicted patient. This patient is most likely to present for care of an infection, accounting for 27.5% of drug-related hospital admissions. The most common infections include cellulitis and the subsequent formation of an abscess at the site of injection (1).

   An abscess is a localized collection of necrotic tissue, bacteria, and white blood cells, usually caused by the seeding of bacteria into a tissue (2). It begins as a focal accumulation of white blood cells in a space created by the breakdown of cellular materials or by the liquefication of necrotic tissue. Later, the abscess may become walled off by highly vascularized connective tissue that serves as a barrier to further spread (2). Enzymatic processes occurring in the abscess result in increased osmotic pressure, drawing water into the area and producing a large amount of pressure outward that increases the risk of bacterial spread along tissue planes or by way of the blood or lymphatic vessels (3).

The abscess can heal only after the pus has been released, since the presence of the pus perpetuates the inflammation. Without surgical intervention, the abscess may heal by proteolytic digestion of the cellular debris which is then resorbed into the blood. Alternately, the fluid may stay loculated in its fibrous capsule to create a cyst or may accumulate calcium salts to become a calcified mass. Most often, the abscess will burrow to the surface of the skin and rupture, thereby releasing the purulent material and causing extensive tissue damage (2). Surgical incision and drainage interrupts this process and is the mainstay of abscess care. Open drainage relieves the pressure inside the cavity; reduces the bacterial number; and, thus, toxin production; and allows the white blood cells to operate efficiently (3).

2. **How is the bacteria introduced into the tissues? Which bacteria are commonly involved?**

The bacteria may be seeded into the tissue by several routes: a contaminated needle or syringe (especially if "works" are shared among intravenous drug users), injection through contaminated skin, contamination of the drug with bacteria or fungi, mixing powdered drugs with an unsterile diluent (e.g., tap water or saliva), or by introducing oral flora when the user blows a blood clot out of a used needle (4).

Only a few studies have been conducted to identify the bacteria commonly involved in abscess formation related to intravenous drug use. These have produced varying results. Bacteria recovered from these abscesses are usually a mix of anaerobes and aerobes, with *Staphylococcus aureus,* β-hemolytic streptococcus, and oral flora predominating (5–7). Results of these studies vary with the geographic area studied. It is important for the practitioner to be aware of the specific bacteria that are frequently recovered from patients in the geographic area in which he or she is working, since antibiotic therapy should be initiated before culture results are known in order to control local cellulitis and bacteremia (6).

A quick and reliable method for determining the types of organisms involved in a specific abscess is the Gram stain. In general, the Gram stain shows one of three patterns: (1) white blood cells without bacteria, indicating a sterile abscess, (2) a mixed pattern of Gram-positive and Gram-negative rods and cocci, indicating a mixed aerobic and anaerobic infection, and (3) Gram-positive cocci in grapelike clusters, diagnostic of *S. aureus.* Additionally, anerobic organisms may produce a characteristic feculent odor, or air may be noted on the x-ray in the tissues surrounding the wound.

3. **What information should the assessment of the patient with a soft tissue abscess include?**

    The history obtained by the nurse practitioner should include (1) the mechanism of injury if it is known, such as intravenous drug use, or a puncture wound to the foot by a nail; (2) in the case of a puncture wound, the material causing the wound, whether wood, metal, or glass, and the possibility of a foreign body in the wound if the material was rusty or was not removed intact; (3) the location of the abscess; (4) the duration and progression of the patient's symptoms; (5) any systemic signs possibly indicative of bacteremia, such as malaise, fever, chills, tachycardia; (6) the possibility of immunocompromise due to HIV infection, renal failure, diabetes or blood dyscrasia; (7) tetanus immunization status; (8) present medications; (9) drug allergies; (10) substance-abuse behaviors; and (11) in the case of substance abuse, readiness for treatment referral.

    The physical examination of the patient should include vital signs; the location and size of the wound in centimeters; the presence of redness, swelling, induration, purulent material, or fluctuance; range of motion of the extremity involved; any vascular or neurological involvement; and the presence of lymphadenopathy or lymphangitis. Diagnostic testing of the patient may include a CBC with differential if the infection is extensive and/or associated with signs of systemic involvement, a needle aspiration at the site of cellulitis if the presence of an abscess is unclear, a wound culture, a radiograph for the presence of subcutaneous air or foreign body if indicated by the mechanism of injury, a Gram stain to aid the initial decision regarding antibiotic therapy, and/or blood cultures if the infection is extensive or associated with signs of systemic involvement.

4. **What is the medical therapy required for this patient?**

    Since the great majority of abscesses do not resolve spontaneously, but go on to burrow through the tissues to the surface causing extensive tissue damage, surgical incision and drainage (I and D) is most important in interrupting this process. Surgical I and D will allow the wound to heal by secondary intention. After I and D, the goal of wound care is to prevent the skin edges from closing prematurely over an unhealed cavity and to cleanse the wound of pus and debris allowing healing to progress. An abscess that extends into the subcutaneous tissues and that is associated with edema or induration will have a cavity after I and D and should be managed by copious irrigation, packed with a dampened gauze wick, and covered with a dry layer of gauze, creating a wet-to-dry dressing which separates the edges of the wound and prevents premature wound closing. This type of wound packing also serves to draw the purulent discharge from the wound by osmotic pressure (8–10). Burney (8) recommends irrigation 2 to 3 times daily and replacement of the wet-to-dry dressing until the wound begins to fill in and no longer produces purulent drainage.

In addition to surgical I and D the use of antibiotics may be required. Usually, in patients with normal host defenses, antibiotics are not needed. However, in the population of intravenous drug users, host defenses are often compromised and antibiotics are necessary. Antibiotics are further indicated in the presence of surrounding erythema and induration, lymphadenopathy or lymphadenitis, and/or systemic symptoms such as malaise, fever, chills, and tachycardia. The antibiotic of choice is determined by knowledge of the organisms commonly isolated from abscesses in the immediate geographic area, the Gram stain, the presence of a feculent odor or of air in the soft tissues as indicated on the x-ray, and by culture and sensitivity testing (9, 10). In the studies previously mentioned, culture and sensitivity tests revealed that penicillin alone covered most of the organisms involved and that a first-generation cephalosporin covered all the organisms involved (5–7). Once antibiotic therapy has been initiated, cellulitis should resolve within 36 to 48 hrs. Tetanus prophylaxis should be updated with a tetanus/diphtheria booster since Tanya did receive the three initial doses as required for school attendance but does not remember receiving a booster within the past 5 years (11).

Effective treatment of these abscesses also involves immobilization, elevation, and heat. If the wound is in a mobile body area such as near a joint, immobilization will help prevent muscle movement from forcing bacteria into the lymphatic or venous systems. Elevation above the level of the heart helps to prevent dependent edema promoting host resistance by maintaining a normal blood supply. Heat increases the blood supply and also helps to localize the infection.

Follow-up is required within 24 hr of initial therapy to monitor resolution of any systemic symptoms or cellulitis and to perform the initial dressing change. Based on this follow-up assessment the provider will determine how the individual patient should be followed. If appropriate, the patient or a family member is taught to provide wound care at home.

5. **What nursing diagnoses apply to this patient?**

   Diagnosis: Anxiety related to the treatment of her illness and the possibility of pain

   Desired patient outcome: The patient will describe a basic understanding of her illness and the treatment involved, and the measures which will be employed to help reduce her pain. The patient will demonstrate a reduction in anxiety; for example, she may cease crying or clenching her fists and assume a more relaxed posture.

   Diagnosis: Pain related to the I and D procedure and subsequent wound care procedures

   Desired patient outcome: The patient will state that her pain is minimized or controlled; the patient will not exhibit nonverbal cues of discomfort.

   Diagnosis: Altered family process related to the patient's poor relationship with her husband

   Desired patient outcome: The patient will begin to formulate a plan to address her dysfunctional relationship in regard to her illness.

   Diagnosis: Impaired skin and tissue integrity related to local infectious process

   Desired patient outcome: The patient's cellulitis will resolve and the abscess will heal without sequela.

   Diagnosis: Disturbance in self-esteem related to the patient's sense of moral failure in abusing drugs

   Desired patient outcome: The patient will verbalize a realistic view of her illness without moral condemnation of self. She will identify strengths and other positive aspects of herself. She will describe ways in which she will assume responsibility for her own health and rehabilitation.

   Diagnosis: Knowledge deficit related to self-care of her wound

   Desired patient outcome: The patient will verbalize an understanding of discharge instructions and give a return demonstration of abscess care.

6. **What nursing intervention is required by this patient?**

   Tanya's fear and anxiety regarding her treatment can be greatly reduced by the nurse's therapeutic use of self. The nurse should spend time with the patient to develop trust and rapport. Procedures should be explained carefully so that the patient is prepared and her fear of the unknown is reduced (12). The cause of the abscess and its treatment and prognosis are described. If possible, the nurse should be at the bedside during the I and D procedure to offer encouragement and support.

The patient's pain should be addressed by the nurse, first assessing the patient's response to pain and then providing an ongoing assessment throughout the ED visit. The patient should be positioned as comfortably as possible, in an area with a comfortable temperature. Analgesics should be administered as ordered by the medical provider prior to the I and D procedure. The nurse should be sensitive to the possible dependency needs of the patient and may determine on an individual basis that therapeutic touch is helpful (12). Tanya should be informed that she can expect her pain to be greatly reduced after the I and D procedure. For pain reduction on return visits during dressing changes, Tanya should be instructed to take an oral analgesic prior to the visit. She should maintain elevation of her arm above the level of her heart and keep her splint on to help control the pain.

The nurse's therapeutic use of self can again be employed to address Tanya's lack of self-esteem. Tanya's self-esteem is enhanced when the nurse is able to communicate esteem and concern for the patient through conversation and behavior. A nonjudgmental approach should be maintained throughout the ED visit. The problem of drug addiction as opposed to moral failure should be distinguished by the nurse for this patient since it seems to be of major concern to her. The nurse can help the patient identify strengths she possesses which will aid her to pursue her recovery. Tanya would benefit from referral to a mental health provider or a drug rehabilitation program that can address her lack of self-esteem.

As with Tanya's lack of self-esteem, her dysfunctional family relationships cannot be adequately addressed during her brief visit to the ED. During this visit it is desirable to help Tanya begin to formulate a plan to deal with the immediate crisis of the effect of her illness on her family relationships. Referral to another source for ongoing care is necessary.

The disruption of Tanya's skin and tissue integrity by the abscess and the I and D procedure itself is best managed through education regarding wound healing and wound care procedures. Tanya and a friend or family member must be taught to continue her wound care at home, and observe the wound for signs and symptoms of worsening infection. A return demonstration by the patient is recommended. If a family member or friend is not available, a visiting nurse referral is made to provide dressing changes. Tanya should be given information regarding analgesics and antibiotics as prescribed. She should also understand the importance of follow-up wound checks and have a written return appointment schedule.

REFERENCES

1. White AG: Medical disorders in drug addicts in two hundred consecutive admissions. *JAMA* 223:1469, 1973.
2. Robbins SL: Pathologic basis of disease. Philadelphia: Saunders, 1984:86.
3. Meislin HW: Soft tissue infections. In: Rosen, ed. Emergency medicine: concepts and clinical practice. Washington, DC: Mosby, 1988:1001–1011.
4. Haller PR: Infections in intravenous drug abusers, what makes them different? *Postgrad Med* 83(4): 95–98, 1988.
5. Orangio GR, Pitlick SD, Della LP, et al: Soft tissue infections in parenteral drug abusers. *Ann Surg* 99(1):97–100, 1984.
6. Biderman P, Hiatt JR: Management of soft tissue infections of the upper extremity in parenteral drug abusers. *Amer J Surg* 154(5):526–528, 1987.
7. Webb D, Thadephalli H: Skin and soft tissue polymicrobial infections from intravenous abuse of drugs. *West J Med* 130(3):200–204, 1979.
8. Burney R: Incision and drainage procedures: soft tissue abscesses in the emergency service. *Emerg Med Clin North Am* 4(3): 527–542, 1986.
9. Meislin HW: Cutaneous abscesses. In: Tintinalli, ed. Emergency medicine: a comprehensive study guide. New York: McGraw-Hill, 1988:663–666.
10. Calia F, Drusano G: Emergency diagnosis and management of infectious disease. In: Schwartz G, ed. Principles and practice of emergency medicine. Philadelphia: Saunders, 1986:1219–1223.
11. Stapczynski SJ: Soft tissue infections. In: Tintinalli S, ed. Emergency medicine: a comprehensive study guide. New York: McGraw-Hill, 1988: 667–669.
12. Rea R, Bourg P, Parker JG, Rushing D: Emergency nursing core curriculum, 3rd ed. Philadelphia: Saunders, 1987: 688–690.

5.2 HUMAN BITE

Suzanne P. Hangasky, RN, BS, CRNP

Lisa is a 15-year-old black female who comes to the ED accompanied by her aunt. She is seeking care for a wound on her left hand and a "bruise" on her right shoulder sustained during an altercation with another teenager 8 hr earlier today. Further questioning reveals that both injuries are human bites. She has done no home wound care. Lisa is a young woman of average stature and build with normal vital signs. There is a puncture wound over the proximal interphalangeal joint of her left middle finger with a small amount of edema and tenderness but no erythema or heat. Lisa has adequate sensation in her finger and hand. There is a 3- by 4-cm ecchymotic region on her right shoulder with tooth imprints at the border but the skin is not punctured. Lisa is unable to remember her tetanus immunization status. She denies past medical problems and any history of allergies or intravenous drug abuse.

Triage Assessment, Acuity Level III: Human bite to the hand over 6 hr old, no distress, wound obvious.

An x-ray of her left finger is obtained and a CBC with differential is sent.

QUESTIONS AND ANSWERS

1. **What are the statistical characteristics of the occurrence of human bite injuries?**

The number of human bites occurring annually is estimated at greater than 60 bites per 100,000 persons (1). Many of these injuries are not evaluated because people are embarrassed about the circumstances surrounding the injury (2). For this same reason, the patient may report the bite as a wound occurring from another type of injury. Those persons who seek early treatment do so because they are concerned about their immunization status or because the wound is serious enough to have developed complications (3).

Most human bites occur as a result of fighting, although self-inflicted bites from thumb sucking, seizures, or falls are reported (1). Forty to seventy-five per cent of human bite injuries involve the hand; other frequent sites are the arms and breasts (1, 4, 5). The incidence of complications is 25 to 50% (1, 5) with the greatest number occurring in bites to the hand. It is interesting to note that the peak incidence of human bite injuries occurs in warm weather and on weekends (1, 6).

2. **What is the pathophysiology resulting from a human bite?**

The human jaw delivers a crushing force, and teeth can cause puncture wounds when a bite occurs. These cause devitalization of tissue and an inoculation of the area with microorganisms from the mouth and skin. When the bite occurs over a clenched fist, the joint is not covered by the dorsal expansion hood and the joint space is easily accessible to puncture. When the finger is extended again, the entrance to the joint may be covered and sealed off. The resulting hypoxic area allows for the proliferation of anerobic organisms. The crushing force delivered may also cause a fracture of the underlying bone. Complications which can develop as a result of the injury include septic arthritis, tendon injury, cellulitis and osteomyelitis. Signs of infection begin in 6 to 12 hrs and spread proximally. The length of time elapsing between injury and treatment is the most important factor in preventing complications (4, 5).

3. **What are the microorganisms most frequently found in human bite injuries?**

The microbiology of the wound is important in the determination of antibiotic therapy for the patient. The bite forces bacteria from the skin and oral cavity into the resulting wound. Normal oral flora, more than skin flora, are found on wound cultures (7). The bacteria grown in cultures from human bite injuries are both aerobic and anaerobic. Frequently found aerobic microorganisms are *Staphylococcus aureus, Eikenella corrodens,* and group A streptococci (3, 7, 8). β-Lactamase activity is noted in 41% of cultures (8). *Eikenella corrodens,* which is present in 20 to 38% of clenched-fist injuries, acts synergistically with α-hemolytic streptococci (6, 8). This polymicrobial combination causes a severe infection which is hard to eradicate.

It is possible to inject viruses and spirochetes with the human bite. Infectious diseases such as hepatitis, scarlet fever, tuberculosis, syphilis, and herpes may be transmitted (3, 6). Since HIV has been found in saliva, in theory, it could be transmitted with a human bite although no cases have been reported (3, 9).

4. **What are the nursing diagnoses for this patient?**

Nursing diagnoses for this patient involve both the injury and the behavior that led to the injury.

Diagnosis: Impaired tissue integrity related to bite injury

Desired patient outcome: The patient will not develop complications of infection, arthritis, osteomyelitis, or cellulitis as evidenced by healing tissue, and absence of drainage, pain, and fever.

Diagnosis: Pain related to tissue ischemia and infection at site of bite injury

Desired patient outcome: The patient will state that there is relief or reduction in pain to the point that it is tolerable. The patient will not exhibit nonverbal cues of pain.

Diagnosis: Impaired social interactions related to emotional response to conflict leading to verbal and physical assault

Desired patient outcome: The patient will describe strategies to avoid or minimize conflict, such as the use of self-control to de-escalate a potentially violent exchange.

Diagnosis: Knowledge deficit related to wound care and importance of follow-up management

Desired patient outcome: The patient will verbalize an understanding of the discharge instructions; the patient will give a return demonstration of correct wound care technique; the patient will state date and time of follow-up appointment and describe how she will arrange to keep the appointment.

5. **What nursing interventions are appropriate for the patient with a human bite injury?**

As with any injured person, the ABCs of assessment should be the first priority. The wounds sustained may be impressive, but the patient must be physiologically stable.

The patient's pertinent history should include how and when the injury occurred, the number of bites sustained, past medical history, and any risk factors that would further increase the potential for wound infection such as diabetes mellitus or immunosuppression. The patient's current immunization status is also needed.

Patient assessment (after the ABCs) should include inspection of each wound. The neurovascular and motor status of all tissue distal to the bite(s) is assessed by looking for the 5 p's: *p*allor, *p*ain, *p*ulselessness, *p*aresthesia, and *p*aralysis. It may be helpful to diagram multiple wounds on a flowchart noting the location and description of each bite: abrasion, laceration, puncture, size, any ecchymosis, edema, erythema, or heat.

A CBC with differential is ordered by the physician and sent to assess any rise in the WBC count that would indicate infection. The x-ray of wounds over bones are ordered to determine if there is any damage to the underlying bone or the presence of any tooth fragment (1, 8, 10).

The need for pain management varies with each patient and is related to the extent and location of the injury and the presence of edema and inflammation. Elevation and functional positioning may reduce the amount of discomfort in an extremity wound. Some patients may require analgesics. If the patient is anxious about her injury, potential procedures, or admission, this may heighten the pain. Reassurance, education, and emotional support throughout the ED visit will help to reduce the level of anxiety.

Wound cleansing is essential. Aggressive management is necessary to prevent infection and to provide good cosmetic and functional results (8). All wounds need to be topically cleansed. Normal saline scrubbing removes most bacteria and does not injure tissue. Other cleansing agents such as 1% povidone-iodine may irritate already damaged tissues. Superficial wounds, such as Lisa's shoulder wound, require no further cleansing (10), but puncture wounds and lacerations (especially those on the hand) require debridement (1, 3, 8). A regional block or other local anesthetic may need to be administered for the procedure. Infected wounds should be cultured. Extremity injuries require immobilization and elevation (1,3). Opinions vary on the need for hospitalization as opposed to outpatient management (2, 5, 9, 10). Considerations include the severity, age, and site of the wound and predicted patient compliance with follow-up care.

Antibiotic therapy is initiated if the wound exhibits any signs of infection or is on the hand, or if the patient has other health problems that put her at risk for complications (9). Prophylactic antibiotic therapy may be used because a human bite is considered to be a contaminated wound. If the patient is to be discharged, the first dose of antibiotic may be given intravenously to obtain a therapeutic level more expediently. Pencillins are the most active agent against oral inoculates although some bacteria are resistant to the drug (8). Penicillinase-resistant antibiotics or a cephalosporin can be given concurrently to cover those bacteria (1, 8). For the penicillin-allergic adult patient, tetracycline or erythromycin are alternatives (1, 3, 9). A combination of amoxicillin and clavulanate potassium is effective for all human bite pathogens (3).

Tetanus diphtheria or toxoid is recommended if the patient has not had a booster in the past 10 years (2, 6). Other immunizations or medications may be ordered by the physician if the biter is known to have a communicable disease.

Patient education is of the utmost importance to assure compliance and an optimal outcome. The patient needs to be instructed in proper administration and side effects of the antibiotics and pain medications prescribed. Signs and symptoms of infection must be taught, immobilization and elevation clearly defined, and any wound care instructions reviewed and demonstrated. Return demonstration is a necessity if there is potential for serious knowledge deficit or noncompliance. The need for follow-up care must be stressed: when, where, and with whom, as well as the complications that may ensue if the wound becomes infected or progresses. All instructions should be specific, in writing, and verbally reviewed.

Lisa was seen by a plastic surgeon in the ED because her hand and finger were involved. He administered a regional block for debridement and exploration of the finger wound. A wound culture was obtained. Lisa's hand was splinted and elevated in a Curtis bag. The shoulder wound was scrubbed with gauze and normal saline. A tetanus diphtheria immunization was administered and an intravenous line initiated for administration of pencillin and a cephalosporin. Because the wound was overlying the joint and showed early signs of infection, Lisa was admitted to the hospital for further antibiotic therapy and observation.

Patient education in the ED was aimed at Lisa's understanding of the potential for complications (i.e., the reason for her admission) and to introduce the concept of problem resolution without physical assault. The discharge teaching plan from the hospital should include the information reviewed above and should also assist Lisa in developing strategies for alternative means of conflict resolution.

REFERENCES

1. Martin LT: Human bites: guidelines for prompt evaluation and treatment. *Postgrad Med* 81:221–223, 1987.
2. Faralli VJ, Sullivan JA: Human bite wounds of the hand. *Okla St Med Assoc J* 79:87–90, 1986.
3. Goldstein EJC, Richwald GA: Human and animal bites. *Am Fam Phys* 36: 101–109, 1987.
4. Dryfus UY, Orthop M, Singer M: Human bites of the hand: A study of one hundred and six patients. *J Hand Surg* 11:884–889, 1985.
5. Peoples E, Boswick JA, Scott FA: Wounds of the hand contaminated by human or animal saliva. *J Trauma* 20: 383–389, 1980.
6. Goldstein EJC: Clenched fist injury infections. *Infect Surg* 7:384–390, 1986.
7. Goldstein EJC, Citron DM, Weild B, et al: Bacteriology of human and animal bite wounds. *J Clin Microbiol* 8:667–672, 1978.
8. Brook I: Microbiology of human and animal bite wounds in children. *Pediatr Infect Dis J* 6:29–32, 1987.

9. Callahan M: Controversies in antibiotic choices for bite wounds. *Ann Emerg Med* 17:107–116, 1988.

10. Taylor GA: Management of human bite injuries of the hand. *Can Med Assoc J* 133:191–192, 1985.

5.3 COMPARTMENT SYNDROME: A "FASCIA-NATING" ISSUE

Sharon A. Childs, RN, BSN, CEN

James, a 44-year-old, mildly retarded, Caucasian male, with a history of hypertension and diabetes mellitus, was brought to the ED by ground ambulance. He had been standing on the street corner waiting to cross when he was struck by a car.

James was designated as a priority 2 case by the paramedics. His Glasgow coma score was rated at 15/15. Peripheral intravenous access with 1000 ml D$_5$/Ringer's lactate was established. Oxygen was provided by non-rebreather mask, and spinal immobilization was initiated. Gross deformity was evident in James' lower extremities. He was unable to move either limb. Pedal pulses were not palpable. James was splinted with two metal, long leg, posterior splints by the paramedics and was immediately brought to the treatment area of the ED for further assessment and treatment.

Triage Assessment, Acuity Level IV: Distal extremity injury, gross injury with cardiovascular and motor deficit.

While in the treatment area of the ED, James' vital signs were BP 180/100, pulse 104, and respirations 24. His lab values were within normal limits. His cardiopulmonary and neurological findings were unremarkable. X-rays revealed positive deformity to both lower extremities. Ecchymosis was present over the proximal tibia. His left foot was warm, with a positive dorsalis pedis pulse by Doppler; his right leg was deformed and tense with an extensive hematoma to the anterior and lateral portions of the leg. Right posterior tibial and dorsalis pedis pulses were obtained by Doppler, but found to be diminished. Right popliteal pulse was absent. James was unable to evert his right ankle. However, sensation was intact to the right peroneal nerve distribution. Left peroneal nerve sensibility was intact.

James was diagnosed as having bilateral proximal tibia and fibula fractures, a right tibial plateau fracture, and a posterior fracture and dislocation of the right knee. The fractured and dislocated right knee was causing occlusion to the right popliteal artery at the level of the knee.

During the assessment, evaluation, and treatment phase in the ED, James was complaining of increasing right lower leg pain. Narcotic analgesia had afforded little relief of his pain. It was becoming evident that the mechanism and extent of injury was precipitating one of the most serious orthopedic complications—compartment syndrome. Compartment pressures were obtained by Wick catheter (1) (Fig. 5.3.1). Anterior compartment pressure was recorded to be 60 mm Hg; superficial posterior compartment pressure was 48 mm Hg. James was immediately prepared and taken to surgery for compartmental decompression fasciotomy, open reduction and internal fixation of fractures, and exploration of the popliteal artery and possible vascular bypass.

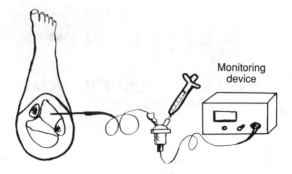

Figure 5.3.1. Insertion of the Wick catheter. (From Pradka L: Use of the Wick catheter for diagnosing and monitoring compartment syndrome. *Orthop Nurs* 4(4):17–18, 1985. Reproduced with permission of the publisher, *Orthopaedic Nursing,* official publication of the National Association of Orthopaedic Nurses.)

QUESTIONS AND ANSWERS

1. What is the pathogenesis of compartment syndrome?

When tissue injury occurs from phenomena such as trauma and burns (thermal or chemical), biochemical changes activate an inflammatory response. At the cellular level, macrophages and neutrophils are stimulated into action. There is also liberation of many tissue products which enhance the inflammatory response. Some of these products include histamine, bradykinin, serotonin, and prostaglandin and reaction by-products from the complement and blood-clotting systems. Damaged vessels in the ischemic muscle dilate from the effects of histamine and these other tissue products. This dilation affects the mean capillary pressure. Hydrostatic filtration pressure becomes greater than the oncotic pressure of the plasma colloids causing plasma proteins and fluid to shift to the interstitium. With the accumulation of fluid in the interstitium, an increase in the hydrostatic pressure inhibits adequate drainage from the venous end of the capillary. The disequilibrium of the pressure gradients within the muscle hinders microvascular perfusion to the tissues. The cycle of edema, increased tissue pressures, and decreased perfusion leads to ischemia with a repetitive sequence until signs and symptoms of compartment syndrome are evident (2–8). Compartment syndrome can be defined as a local condition in which edematous and ischemic muscle is confined within an osteofascial compartment (Fig. 5.3.2).

TIP: Fracture of the lateral condyle or plateau of the tibia is a result of blunt trauma to the lateral aspect of the knee. While the feet remain in a planted and fixed position, severe abductive valgus strain is placed upon the knee resulting in subluxation or complete dislocation of the joint (9). This type of injury is commonly referred to as a "bumper fracture" and frequently results in compartment syndrome.

Bleeding into tissues that occurs from a contusion, fracture, or other injury also acts like a foreign body stimulating the inflammatory response (2). Other causes of compartment syndrome are direct arterial vascular insult (occlusion), constricting bandages, casts, fractures, infections, and insect and animal bites (8, 10). Prolonged limb compression results in an interrelated problem: compartment syndrome and crush syndrome (11, 12). Signs and symptoms associated with compartment syndrome are described in Table 5.3.1. Tissue necrosis, nerve damage, and paralysis are sequelae of compartment syndrome.

Systemic evidence of muscle necrosis can include myoglobinuria, renal failure, acidosis, and hyperkalemia with resultant cardiac involvement (12, 13). Unless intervention to release the pressure is promptly instituted, tamponade of perfusion to the tissues will result in muscle and nerve ischemia which will cause permanent and irreparable damage.

2. **What nursing diagnoses are relevant to this case?**
   The patient who has sustained significant soft tissue injury is a candidate for developing neurovascular compromise. The following are the pertinent nursing diagnoses for this patient.

   Diagnosis: Pain related to muscle ischemia, fracture, and neurovascular compromise

   <u>Desired patient outcome:</u>   The patient will describe relief of or experience significant reduction in the sensation of pain.

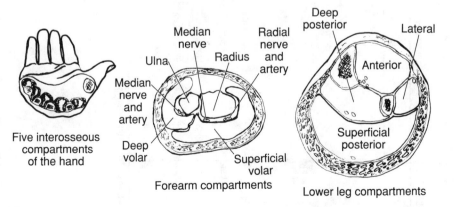

Figure 5.3.2.   Extremity osteofacial compartments.

Table 5.3.1 Associated Signs and Symptoms Seen in Compartment Syndrome

Compartment	Areas of Sensibility Deprivation	Muscular Motor Weakness	Pain on Passive Flexion or Extension	Region of Muscle Tenseness
Forearm				
Dorsal	None	Extension of wrist and fingers	Flexion of wrist and fingers	Dorsal forearm
Volar	Ulnar and median nerve distribution on palm side of fingers	Flexion of wrist and fingers	Extension of wrist and fingers	Volar forearm
Hand				
Interosseous	None	Interosseous muscles	Abduction and adduction of the metacarpal joints	Dorsum of hand between metacarpal joints
Lower leg				
Anterior	Web space of great toe	Toe extensors and tibialis anterior	Toe flexion	Anterior aspect of tibia
Lateral	Dorsum of foot	Peroneal muscles	Inversion of foot	Lateral aspect of lower leg
Superficial posterior	None	Soleus and gastrocnemius	Dorsiflexion of foot	Calf of leg
Deep posterior	Sole of foot	Toe flexors and tibialis posterior	Toe extension	Distal midportion of leg between Achilles tendon and area of tibia

From Matsen FA: Compartment syndrome: A unified concept. *Clin Orthop Relat Res* 113:8–14, 1975; Copyright JB Lippincott (Harper & Row).

Diagnosis: Alteration in peripheral tissue perfusion related to localized tissue edema; obstruction of microvascular circulation causing compromised neurovascular status

Desired patient outcome: The patient will maintain normal compartment pressures as evidenced by compartmental readings of 20 mm Hg or less; the patient will regain distal pulses, have reduction in lower extremity pain, and report decreased numbness and tingling.

Diagnosis: Impaired mobility related to multiple fractures

Desired patient outcome: The patient will be free of preventable complications of immobility (e.g., pneumonia, decubiti, and renal calculi); the patient will perform mobilization activities with assistance.

Diagnosis: Impaired tissue integrity related to fractures, fasciotomies, and surgical wounds

Desired patient outcome: The patient will have normal progress of tissue healing evidenced by clean wound and pink, healthy tissue.

Diagnosis: Potential for infection related to impaired tissue integrity

Desired patient outcome: The patient will not experience signs or symptoms of infection as evidenced by temperature < 100.4°F; wound drainage will not be odoriferous.

Diagnosis: Knowledge deficit related to limited understanding of treatment modalities, and mild mental retardation

Desired patient outcome: The patient will describe a basic understanding of treatments; the patient will demonstrate the ability to follow instructions related to the treatment plan.

3. **What nursing interventions are appropriate in this case?**

Nursing interventions in James' case as well as for all patients who are suspect for developing musculo-neurovascular compromise (compartment syndrome) focus primarily on astute neurovascular assessment.

TIP: Pain that is unrelieved by narcotic analgesia and expressed as being continual and unrelenting or pain that is elicited by *passive* stretch of the muscles in the involved compartment is pathognomonic for compartment syndrome.

The nurse assesses the patient's neurovascular status by evaluating the five p's: pain, paralysis, paresthesia, pulselessness, and pallor. *Pain* is assessed for its location, type (burning, stabbing, aching, throbbing), intensity, duration, and precipitating or aggravating variables such as position or temperature change (cold). *Paralysis* can be evidenced by the patient's inability to flex and extend or invert and evert the affected extremity. *Paresthesia* is a decreased sensibility or described sensation of numbness, tingling, or feeling of pins and needles. *Pulselessness,* a late and detrimental sign, is usually not seen in early compartment syndrome. *Pallor* indicates inadequate arterial perfusion. Cyanosis is indicative of poor venous return (14).

Assessments of the neurological status of the upper and lower extremities are performed by the nurse. Table 5.3.2 illustrates the assessment criteria.

Vascular assessment is performed by using the Doppler for pulse assessment, checking nail beds for capillary refill time (brisk, diminished, absent), and evaluating temperature (warm, cool, cold) and appearance (pink, cyanotic, pallor, mottled) of the skin (5, 7).

4. **What are the medical interventions that have related nursing implications?**

The medical intervention that is commonly used to detect increased pressure in the affected compartment is intracompartmental pressure monitoring. The procedure is useful in detecting subtle pressure changes even in those persons who because of communication problems (aphasia, comatose, intoxication) or paralysis are not cognizant of the impending situation (4).

Several techniques are available to measure and monitor compartment pressures. Techniques include needle manometer, the Slit catheter, Wick catheter, and the solid-state transducer intracompartmental (STIC) pressure monitor system (1, 4, 15–17). The basic concept for all these methods is the detection of increased pressure within the tissue compartment.

Nursing responsibilities include assisting with insertion of the monitoring device, maintenance of the system while it is inserted, and monitoring of the readings if continuous pressure monitoring is ordered (1). Pain will be relieved by pharmacological and nonpharmacological interventions. Providing physical support and patient comfort by means of chemical analgesia (giving medication and observing the effects), patient positioning, and the nurse's therapeutic use of self (touch and verbal communication) are all important (1, 4, 17–19).

Continued neurovascular assessment in conjunction with the measurement of compartment pressures with accurate documentation of findings is crucial in the care of the patient who is being monitored for compartment syndrome. Untoward changes should be reported to the physician immediately.

Table 5.3.2 Assessment Criteria for Neurological Status

Nerves	Sensory[a]	Motor[b]
	Upper Extremity	
Radial	Test for sensation at the dorsal web space of the thumb. Rationale: Radial nerve discrimination is assessed by this area of sensibility in the hand.	Have patient hyperextend wrist and/or hyperextend thumb. Rationale: Inability to perform strong movement is indicative of potential radial nerve injury. When the radial nerve is significantly damaged, ½ to ¾ of the hand's power is lost.
Ulnar	Test for sensation on the volar (palmar) surface of the tip of fifth (small) finger. Rationale: Ulnar nerve discriminately assessed for in this area of the hand.	Have patient abduct fingers. Rationale: Motor capability necessary for normal hand functioning; pinching.
Median	Test for sensation in the volar (palmar) surface at the tip of the index (second finger). Rationale: Integrity for main sense of touch to hand is elicited here.	Have patient consecutively oppose each finger of hand to the thumb. Rationale: Median nerve is the main nerve of precise functioning (pronation of the hand).
	Lower Extremity	
Peroneal	Test sensation at dorsal web space of first (great) and second toes. Rationale: Nerve innervation can be precisely assessed in this area.	Ask patient to dorsiflex ankle/foot. Rationale: Motor functioning is assessed in this one maneuver.
Tibial	Test sensation to the sole of the foot. Rationale: Sensibility is discriminately assessed in this area.	Ask patient to plantarflex foot. Rationale: Tibial nerve integrity gauged by ability to plantarflex.
Femoral	Test for sensation on the anterior thigh. Rationale: Nerve innervation best assessed on anterior thigh.	Have patient do straight leg raise. Rationale: Motor functioning interrupted if unable to straight leg raise because of decreased power.

[a]Sensibility is graded as normal, numbness, tingling, diminished, or absent sensation.
[b]Motor ability is classified as normal, decreased, or absent.

Compartment pressures of 0 to 20 mm Hg are normal; pressures of 21 to 30 mm Hg are indicative of insidious compartment syndrome (decreased microvascular perfusion), and pressures greater than 40 mm Hg indicate compartment syndrome (ischemic necrosis).

TIP: *Do not elevate extremity.* Elevation above the level of the heart is contraindicated because venous drainage is already impeded because of edema. Elevation would further decrease arterial perfusion and increase ischemia.

When compartment pressures exceed 30 to 40 mm Hg, decompression fasciotomy of the affected compartment is performed. Unless the patient is in extremis, the nurse will prepare the patient for the operating room (OR), attending to the usual preoperative checklist activities and making sure the physician has explained the need for surgery and the procedure to the patient. Offering emotional support to the patient as well as providing good preoperative teaching will expedite the patient's postoperative course.

After the fasciotomy, the nurse's dynamic role in continued neurovascular assessment is necessary. Postfasciotomy complications are prevented by continued assessment of the wound, observing for local and systemic signs and symptoms of developing infection, and following the medical regimen, including dressings, antibiotics, and pressure monitoring as indicated.

REFERENCES

1. Pradka L: Use of the Wick catheter for diagnosing and monitoring compartment syndrome. *Orthop Nurs* 4(4):17–18, 1985.
2. Guyton A: Textbook of medical physiology. 7th ed. Philadelphia: Saunders, 1986.
3. Matsen F: Compartment syndrome: A unified concept. *Clin Orthop* 113:8–15, 1975.
4. Proehl J: Compartment syndrome. *J Nurs* 14(5):283–292, 1988.
5. Conry K, Bies C: Compartment syndrome: A complication of intra-aortic balloon pump. *Dimens Crit Care Nurs* 4(5):274–284, 1985.
6. Carrieri V, Lindsey A, West C: Pathophysiological phenomenon in nursing: Human responses to illness. Philadelphia: Saunders, 1986.
7. Callahan J: Compartment syndrome. *Orthop Nurs* 4(4):11–15, 1985.
8. Rorabeck C, Macnab I: The pathophys-

iology of anterior tibial compartment syndrome. *Clin Orthop* 113:52–57, 1975.
9. Salter R: Textbook of disorders and injuries of the musculoskeletal system. Baltimore: Williams & Wilkins, 1970.
10. Patman R: Compartment syndrome in peripheral vascular surgery. *Clin Orthop* 113:103–110, 1975.
11. Mubarak S, Hargens A: Compartment syndrome and Volkmann's contracture. Philadelphia: Saunders, 1981.
12. Mubarak S, Owen C: Compartment syndrome and its relation to the crush syndrome: A spectrum disease. *Clin Orthop* 113:81–89, 1975.
13. Oman K: Sequelae to ruptured aortic aneurysm. *Crit Care Nurse* 5(6):14–19, 1985.
14. Farrell J: Illustrated guide to orthopedic nursing. 3rd ed. New York: Lippincott, 1986.
15. Whitesides T, Haney T, Morimoto K,

Harada H: Tissue pressure measurements as a determinant for the need of fasciotomy. *Clin Orthop* 113:43–51, 1975.

16. Kuska B: Acute onset of compartment syndrome. *J Emerg Nurs* 8(2):75–79, 1982.

17. Larson M, Leigh J, Wilson L: Detecting compartment syndrome using continuous pressure monitoring. *Focus Crit Care* 13(5):51–56, 1986.

18. Dossey B, Keegan L, Guzzetta C, Kolkmeir L: Holistic nursing: handbook for practice. Rockville, MD: Aspen Publishers, 1988.

19. Kenner C, Guzzetta C, Dossey B: Critical Care Nursing: Body-Mind-Spirit. 2nd ed. Boston: Little, Brown, 1985.

5.4 HYPOTHERMIA: A WINTER EMERGENCY

Cathy Robey-Williams, RN, MS, CCRN

Jason and his friends were walking home from basketball practice when they noticed a bonfire on the frozen river. A few of their friends were out in the middle ice-skating. When walking with his friends toward the bonfire to socialize, Jason fell through the ice. The rest of the group stood frozen with fear. When Jason did not return to the surface, one of his friends ran to shore and called 911 from the closest house.

The first emergency unit to arrive on the scene was an engine crew who placed a ladder on the ice out to the hole near the bonfire. The fire was extinguished and the other teens instructed to return to shore following the ladder. Ten minutes later rescue divers arrived and began their search pattern. After 12 min, Jason was brought to the surface. Basic life support was begun as Jason was slid back to shore. He was immediately placed into the awaiting helicopter and orally intubated with a no. 8 endotracheal tube. The flight to the closest trauma center took 3 min. During that time Jason's wet clothing was removed and he was wrapped in a blanket.

The ED was alerted that a 16-year-old male weighing an estimated 80 kg had fallen through the ice. The patient would be arriving in full cardiac arrest, intubated with basic cardiac life support initiated. The ED's resuscitation team was alerted and began to prepare for the child's arrival. The OR staff were also notified.

Triage Assessment, Acuity Level IV: Cardiopulmonary arrest and profound hypothermia.

Upon arrival to the ED, basic life support is continued. Heated humidified oxygen is initiated via ambu bag. Two large bore intravenous lines are started, and warmed NS is infused at a temperature of 40°C via a rapid warmer-infuser device. Jason's initial rectal temperature was 26.6°C. During the first 15 min of the resuscitation effort Jason has an additional 2°C drop in temperature. A nasogastric tube is passed and warm NS lavages begun. Urethral and rectal Foley catheters are introduced and warm NS enemas initiated. Several doses of epinephrine are administered, without response from the heart. Jason is therefore taken to the OR and placed on heart-lung bypass. After his blood is warmed to 32.2°C, an idioventricular rhythm is noted via ECG. Epinephrine increases the rate to 40 beats per minute. Jason is maintained on bypass until his temperature reaches 35.5°C. At that time Jason's HR is 62, BP 100/60, and he is mechanically ventilated. He is then transferred to the intensive care unit for continued monitoring.

QUESTIONS AND ANSWERS

1. **What effects does rapid immersion hypothermia have on the major body systems?**

    Central blood temperature receptors located in the anterior hypothalamus compare core body temperature to messages received regarding peripheral or shell body temperature. As blood circulating to the brain cools, the hypothalamus sends messages to the adrenal medulla to release catecholamines and directs neural pathways to vasoconstrict. The hypothalamus can also stimulate the body to shiver which can produce the same amount of heat as maximum exercise for limited periods of time (1). These compensatory mechanisms are usually effective during normal cycles of temperature change such as going outdoors during the winter months. When these compensatory mechanisms are ineffective, such as during intense or prolonged exposure to cold, the brain cools and cerebral O_2 consumption decreases. Cerebral blood flow then decreases and sludging and a decreased level of consciousness occur. At a core body temperature below 30°C consciousness is lost, reflexes decrease, pupils dilate, and the body lies in a near dormant state.

    The respiratory system also attempts to compensate during cooling. Bronchodilation occurs and the oxygen-hemoglobin dissociation curve shifts to the left. Cessation of breathing occurs at temperatures around 24°C. The GI tract becomes silent at a temperature of 35°C. The genitourinary tract is affected by an increase in serum glucose as the sympathetic nervous system is stimulated, thus causing the adrenal glands to secrete catecholamines. Elevated serum glucose combined with inadequate levels of insulin produces glucose excretion in the urine and a concomitant diuresis of fluid (1).

    The cardiovascular system is the primary organ system affected by hypothermia. Cooling of Purkinje fibers below 25°C decreases resting transmembrane potential, depresses action potential height, slows conduction velocity, prolongs absolute and relative refractory periods, and slows the rate of spontaneous depolarization. In humans cooled for cardiac surgery, ventricular fibrillation occurs at 23°C and asystole occurs at 20°C (2).

    Metabolic changes that occur during hypothermia include depletion of body stores of fat, carbohydrates, and protein; stimulation of catecholamines and glucocorticoids; reduction in insulin activity; and reduction in liver function secondary to inhibition of the enzyme hexokinase. Initially hypothermia causes a shift of fluid to the extracellular compartment and induces diuresis creating relative hypovolemia. At temperatures below 25°C water moves into the cells and fluid is sequestered in the capillaries which results in hemoconcentration and increased blood viscosity (3, 4). Prolonged clotting times are evident at 20°C. Leukopenia and thrombocytopenia also occur and are a result of sequestration of cells in the liver and spleen (4). Table 5.4.1 correlates temperature and clinical manifestations of hypothermia.

2. **Why was advanced life support delayed in the field and initiated only after arrival to the ED?**

Until the central body organs are rewarmed, pharmacological and electrical therapy are ineffective. In fact, giving cardiac arrest drugs to a hypothermic patient can be deleterious. As the body rewarms, the drugs that have been dormant because of the cold state are then activated and begin affecting the body concurrently. At 28°C the heart rate slows to 50% of normal. Between 20 and 28°C the heart rate drops down to 20% of normal until asystole occurs, usually at 20°C. The risk of dysrhythmias increases after temperatures drop below 28°C. This is due to decreased flow to the myocardium secondary to

Table 5.4.1 Correlation between Temperature and Clinical Symptoms

Temperature, °C	Clinical Manifestations
35–37	Cold sensation
	Moderate shivering
	Loss of coordination
32–35	Violent shivering
	Slurred speech
	Confusion
	Amnesia
	Tachycardia
	Vasoconstriction
28–32	Decreased shivering
	Muscle rigidity
	Bradycardia
	Atrial fibrillation
	Cyanosis
	Hypoventilation
	Systemic lactic acidosis
25–28	Hypotension
	Stupor
	Coma
	Irregular pulse
	Ventricular fibrillation if heart stimulated
	Cold diuresis
21–25	Spontaneous ventricular fibrillation
	Areflexia
	Pupils fixed, dilated
	No spontaneous movement
	Apnea
	Asystole

From Johnston JB: Hypothermia: assessment and intervention. *Emerg Nurs Rep* 3(8):5, 1988. Reprinted with permission of Aspen Publishers, Inc., © November 1988.

vasoconstriction and viscosity of blood. Ventricular fibrillation is a common complication during this time precipitated by hypocapnia, alkalosis, rewarming (especially surface rewarming), and physical manipulation of the heart. Sometimes movement of the victim's body or endotracheal intubation will stimulate ventricular fibrillation (2, 4). Ventricular fibrillation is resistant to defibrillation and antiarrythmic drugs below a core temperature of 28°C (5).

3. **What other situations could lead to hypothermia?**

The definition of hypothermia is a core temperature that is less than 35°C. Heat loss occurs through four physical mechanisms. Conduction is heat lost through direct contact. An example is heat lost through contact with water. The thermal conductivity of water is 30 times greater than that of air, which is why cold water immersion is so devastating to the body. Convection is heat transfer by movement. An example is heat lost by wind blowing against the body and disrupting the warmed air surrounding the body. Radiation is heat lost through the skin, for example, the unprotected head. Evaporation is heat lost through warm fluid loss. Examples are heat lost from a burn patient due to plasma excretion through the skin or heat losses from the respiratory tract during ventilation.

The physical mechanisms of heat loss are easily understood in situations of exposure to harsh weather or immersion hypothermia as in Jason's case. These type of situations are encountered more frequently in rural areas as a result of accidents during outdoor activities. A more complex problem is that of urban hypothermia, characterized by chronic generalized cooling of highly susceptible individuals (6).

Individuals with impaired thermoregulatory systems are prone to hypothermia and do not require exposure to severe cold to experience heat loss. The most significant high-risk population is the elderly (7). An epidemiological study of deaths as a result of hypothermia found the highest risk group to be those 85 years of age and over. Comparing demographic data for the entire population over 65 years of age, more nonwhites died of hypothermia regardless of sex, and more men died of hypothermia regardless of color. The same study evaluated Washington D.C. statistics and found that out of all the people who died from hypothermia in 1982, 50% had elevated blood alcohol levels, 50% had inadequate housing, and 30% were malnourished (8).

Rationales for the high risk of the elderly population are consistently reported throughout the literature. These risks include decreased peripheral sensation to cold, functional disability, poverty, and social isolation (6–10). Other populations at risk for hypothermia are those with underlying diseases that impair normal thermoregulation. Examples are patients experiencing shock (hypovolemic, cardiogenic, neurogenic), Gram-negative sepsis, staphylococcal pneumonia, hypoendocrine states (thyroid, adrenal, pituitary), profound anemia, pulmonary edema, acute renal failure, epidural hematoma, seizures, hypoglycemia, hypothalamic and CNS dysfunction [Wernicke's encephalopathy, head trauma, tumor, cerebrovascular accident (CVA)], and dermal disease (burns, exfoliative dermititis).

Patients who arrive to the ED for primary illnesses as listed above may, upon further examination, be found to be hypothermic. Conversely, patients brought to the department because of hypothermia may have an underlying condition that prohibits normal response to warming treatment.

Chronic hypothermia occurs gradually with subtle heat losses over time. In most cases the individual does not realize the loss is occurring and therefore does not take action. Patients in social isolation are at greatest risk because no one is aware that cooling is taking place. The individual eventually becomes less active, and neurological function is impaired. Patients in this circumstance are often rescued by concerned neighbors, family, or friends that have not heard nor seen the individual for extended periods of time.

Intoxication with alcohol is the most common cause of urban hypothermia. However, with increasing drug use, hypothermia can also be anticipated in patients with overdoses from cocaine and heroin. Alcohol as a vasodilator increases heat loss to the environment as well as depresses normal CNS temperature control function. In addition to alcohol and illicit drugs there are also several groups of medications that directly interfere with normal thermoregulatory mechanisms predisposing some consumers to hypothermia (8). These medications include nicotine, neuroleptics (tubocurarine, pancuronium), phenothiazines, tricyclic antidepressants, benzodiazapines, narcotics, reserpine, barbiturates, and β-blockers.

Another population of patients often overlooked that is predisposed to altered sensorium or inability to respond to the cold are patients with psychiatric disorders such as acute psychosis and profound depression (10). The pediatric patient population especially neonates are also at risk for hypothermia regardless of weather conditions. Air-conditioned treatment rooms can pose a major threat to a newborn if the infant is not properly dried, wrapped, and placed in a warm environment. Premature infants with little or no subcutaneous fat, underdeveloped neurological systems with inability to shiver, and large body surface area lose heat quickly. In fact, infant core body temperatures drop immediately upon delivery and require immediate measures to replace heat loss. Hypothermia in neonates results in a cascade of events which can lead to hypoglycemia, seizures, and death.

4. **What nursing diagnoses are appropriate for this case?**

Nursing diagnoses related to the management of Jason's hypothermia and cardiopulmonary arrest are essential. If Jason survives, he and his family will require instruction on identification and management of future potential medical problems related to complications of hypothermia and treatment as well as safety measures that will prevent this sort of accident from happening again.

Diagnosis: Hypothermia related to accidental cold water immersion for 30 min

<u>Desired patient outcome:</u> The patient's core body temperature will increase to normothermia in response to active core rewarming interventions.

Diagnosis: Ineffective breathing pattern related to absence of CNS function

<u>Desired patient outcome:</u> Artificial ventilation will provide the patient with symmetrical chest expansion; the patient will have breath sounds, heard in all lung fields.

Diagnosis: Impaired gas exchange related to decreased oxygen delivery from cardiopulmonary arrest and pulmonary edema secondary to fresh water drowning

<u>Desired patient outcome:</u> The patient will maintain a $PaO_2 \geq$ 90 to 100 mm Hg and maintain capillary oxygen saturation above 97%; the patient will have clear breath sounds, pink mucous membranes, and brisk capillary refill.

Diagnosis: Decreased cardiac output related to cardiac arrest secondary to hypothermia

<u>Desired patient outcome:</u> The patient will have normal cardiac function following rapid core rewarming of the heart evidenced by ECG showing sinus rhythm, systolic $BP \geq 90$ mm Hg, $HR \leq$ 100 beats/min; urinary output ≥ 30 ml/hr.

Diagnosis: Fluid volume deficit related to vasodilation and diuresis of intravascular volume

<u>Desired patient outcome:</u> The patient will maintain a systolic $BP \geq 90$ mm Hg, $HR \leq 100$ beats/min, and urinary output ≥ 30 ml/hr.

Diagnosis: Altered cardiopulmonary tissue perfusion related to hypothermia

<u>Desired patient outcome:</u> The patient will respond to core rewarming by converting asystole to a perfusing rhythm and upon reaching normothermia will maintain a sinus rhythm. The patient's ECG will show no PVCs nor evidence of myocardial isch-

emia (absence of J waves, ST elevation, ST depression, or inverted T waves).

Diagnosis: *Altered cerebral tissue perfusion related to hypothermia*
Desired patient outcome: The patient will respond to core rewarming by return of neurological function as evidenced by pupils constricting briskly to light, return of reflexes, response to stimuli, and response to verbal commands.

Diagnosis: *Knowledge deficit related to accidental cold water immersion via fall through ice*
Desired patient outcome: The patient will be able to describe risks associated with walking on ice. The patient will describe proper actions to take if confronted with the same situation in the future. The patient will identify emergency measures that should be taken if he is witness to a similar incident.

5. **What are the appropriate nursing interventions for Jason?**

Figures 5.4.1 and 5.4.2 describe the standard algorithm for management of hypothermia. As the algorithm describes, field treatment and initial ED treatment for cases like Jason focus on airway, breathing, and circulation. The nurse caring for Jason must ensure airway patency by assessing the placement of the endotracheal tube, chest expansion, and breath sounds. A heating unit placed around an oxygen humidifier prior to patient arrival will provide for heated 100% oxygen delivery to the patient. Optimal gas exchange can be ensured by the nurse's vigilant suctioning of excess secretions and continuous monitoring and reporting of the patient's oxygenation status.

Nursing interventions related to cardiovascular function follow the primary goal of returning the patient's core body temperature to normal. Extracorporeal blood rewarming if available is considered the best treatment for patients like Jason in cardiopulmonary arrest with temperatures below 28°C (1, 10–13). This is accomplished by gaining vascular access to the femoral artery and vein and circulating the patient's blood through the bypass machine until core temperature reaches 30 to 32°C. Disadvantages to this technique include the need for special equipment, the need for an OR team and a perfusionist, the heparinized state of the patient, potential damage to red blood cells, and potential damage to blood vessels.

Other methods of active core body rewarming include intragastric balloon inflation, colonic irrigation, mediastinal irrigation, hemodialysis, and peritoneal dialysis. Intragastric balloon inflation is accomplished by passing a cuffed tube down the esophagus until it reaches the stomach. Once placement in the stomach is verified, heated NS is instilled and the cuff is inflated to keep the solution in place. Colonic irrigation is accomplished by inserting a large Foley catheter into the

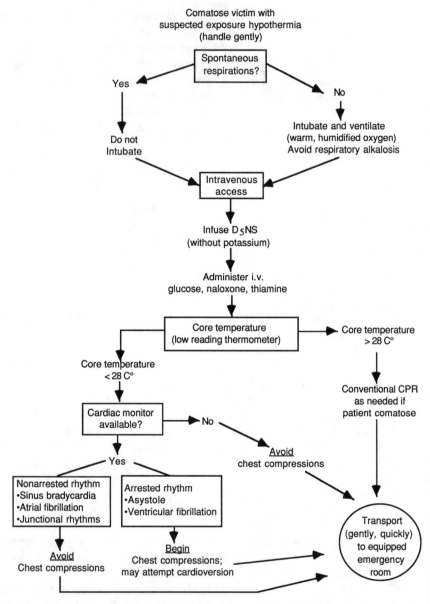

Figure 5.4.1. Prehospital algorithm. (From Zell SC, Kurtz KJ: Severe exposure hypothermia: a resuscitation protocol. *Ann Emerg Med* 14(4): 340, 1985.)

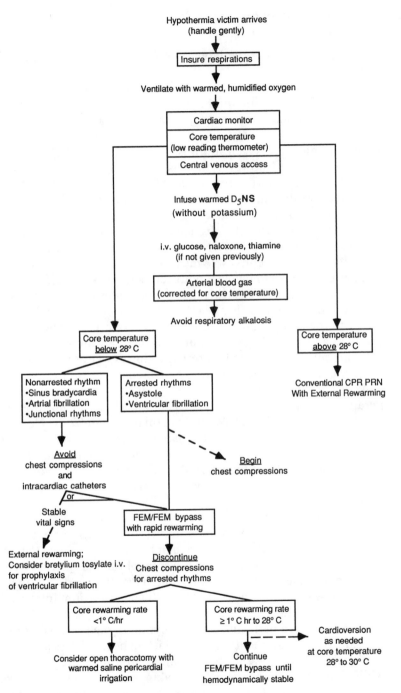

Figure 5.4.2. Emergency department algorithm. (From Zell SC, Kurtz KJ: Severe exposure hypothermia: a resuscitation protocol. *Ann Emerg Med* 14(4): 342, 1985.)

141

rectum and irrigating the large bowel by means of warmed saline enemas.

Mediastinal irrigation is performed after thoracotomy with warmed saline irrigation fluid poured into the chest cavity. Hemodialysis and peritoneal dialysis are performed as usual with attention to maintaining the temperature of the dialysate at 40°C (1, 10, 13). Heated humidified oxygen administration is promoted in most of the literature reviewed; however, there is conflicting evidence as to its effectiveness as a true core rewarmer (11, 12, 14, 15). All these procedures require the emergency nurse to be knowledgeable about the equipment needed, to understand the steps of each technique in order to anticipate and assist the physician as necessary, and to be able to coordinate simultaneous activities while guarding patient safety.

In situations where invasive measures are being used for rewarming, basic measures to increase body temperature should not be overlooked. The nurse, by ensuring that the patient is dry and on a warm surface, will prevent further heat loss. Ensuring that all fluids in contact with the patient have been warmed is essential, including blood products and crystalloids. The nurse must closely monitor and document amounts of fluid used for resuscitation as well as urinary output to ensure that adequate volume is delivered.

As discussed earlier, cardiac arrest drugs are not indicated for temperatures below 28 to 30°C. Several authors (1, 5, 10), however, suggest administering 25 g $D_{50}W$, 100 mg thiamine, and 2 mg Narcan as soon as intravenous access is available. Baseline neurological function as well as response to these medications are important parameters for the nurse to be monitoring. Anticipating for these drugs and having them prepared prior to patient arrival eliminates delay in administration.

Bretylium is one antiarrythmic drug that has been helpful in some hypothermic patients. In one case study (16), 10 mg of bretylium per kg of body weight converted ventricular fibrillation at a core temperature of 29.5°C after 6 min. When the epinephrine was ineffective, the emergency nurse caring for Jason could have suggested to the physician team leader that a dose of 400 to 800 mg bretylium intravenous push might be effective.

When there is a perfusing cardiac rhythm in the presence of hypothermia, the management of the patient can be much less aggressive. The goal of therapy would be to maintain normal cardiac function while gently rewarming the patient, taking care not to stimulate ventricular fibrillation. At temperatures above 30°C rapid rewarming is rarely necessary. Passive methods such as heated humidified oxygen, warm intravenous fluids, and use of an external heat source are usually sufficient (10).

If Jason's case had been less serious and he had been easily warmed in the ED, the nurse would then have to talk with him and his parents to prevent this kind of accident from happening again. Topics for discussion should include making correct choices, how to handle peer pressure, proper actions to take when around ice, methods to protect one's self against heat loss, and how to contact emergency medical services when needed.

6. **After the patient is rewarmed, what complications should be anticipated?**

There are three major groups of complications resulting from active rewarming of a patient: (1) afterdrop, (2) rewarming shock and associated complications from external rewarming, and (3) direct pathology to organ systems from the hypothermic event. There are also complications associated with the various treatment measures as already discussed in question 5.

Afterdrop is defined as a continued fall in body temperature after rewarming maneuvers have been initiated (17). Usually body temperatures will continue to fall during the first 10 to 30 min of resuscitation. This phenomenon occurs primarily with rapid immersion cooling, and rarely with gradual cooling as experienced by the elderly (17). Afterdrop can be minimized by core rewarming, but must be closely monitored during initial resuscitation.

External rewarming of the skin and extremities can have serious negative effects. As the peripheral tissues are warmed, vascular beds dilate, releasing cold acidotic blood to the heart. Rewarming acidosis occurs from circulation of peripheral blood that had become stagnate without flow, resulting in anaerobic metabolism and lactic acid production. Acidosis also occurs as a result of increased metabolic demands of the newly heated peripheral tissues not being met by the cold core body organs (10). This influx of acidotic blood could stimulate the heart into ventricular fibrillation. Dilation of the blood vessels also reduces systemic vascular resistance decreasing blood pressure and further depressing cardiac function (4). Ventricular fibrillation is a common complication during rewarming efforts with patients in initial reperfusion rhythms. This is due to the heart's decreased fibrillatory threshold that is easily triggered by resuscitation procedures. Ventricular fibrillation has been stimulated in patients with temperatures less than 28°C by movement of their body during transit, endotracheal intubation, central line insertion, and introduction of gastric tubes (4, 10, 11).

Even when quick central core rewarming techniques are used, hypothermia continues to have associated complications. Hypoglycemia occurs as a result of depletion of body stores of glucose and is complicated by impaired insulin function (4). Hypovolemia occurs as a result of the shift of body fluids to the extracellular compartment and induced diuresis (3).

Intravascular thrombus formation with MI and CVA is a result of the increase viscosity of the blood that results from massive diuresis. Pneumonia and pulmonary edema are pulmonary insults associated with hypothermia. Other effects of hypothermia include pancreatitis, acute tubular necrosis, alkalosis as a result of K+ excretion, hemolysis, depressed bone marrow activity, disseminated intravascular coagulation, hypophosphatemia, seizures, hematuria, myoglobinuria, temporary adrenal insufficiency, and gastric erosion and hemorrhage (1).

In this case, Jason suffered the worst type of hypothermic insult. In addition, he sustained complications from near drowning in fresh water. According to the National Institutes of Health (7), the chances for a complete recovery are good when core body temperatures do not drop below 32.2°C and there are no other complications. If body temperatures fall between 26.6 and 32.2°C, most victims will recover but may sustain permanent damage. Victims of severe hypothermia with core body temperatures less than 26.6°C have poor chances of survival. Improved systems of patient evacuation and transportation to facilities with advanced technology, coupled with improvements in medical and nursing management of the hypothermic patient, will increase the probability for survival of patients like Jason in the future.

REFERENCES

1. Sivertson KT: Hypothermia. A lecture presented to emergency medicine residents, The Johns Hopkins University School of Medicine, February 24, 1989.
2. Southwick FS, Dalglish PH: Recovery after prolonged asystolic cardiac arrest in profound hypothermia. *JAMA* 243 (12):1250–1253, 1980.
3. Chernow B, Lake CR, Zaritsky A, et al: Sympathetic nervous system "switch off" with severe hypothermia. *Crit Care Med* 11(9):677–679, 1983.
4. Wong KC: Physiology and pharmacology of hypothermia. *West J Med* 138(2): 227–232, 1983.
5. Carden D, Doan L, Sweeney PJ, et al: Hypothermia. *Ann Emerg Med* 11(9): 79–85, 1982.
6. Slovis CM, Bachvarov HL: Heated in-

halation treatment of hypothermia. *Amer J Emerg Med* 2(6):535–536.
7. United States Department of Health and Human Services. Accidental hypothermia. Pamphlet produced by The National Institutes of Health, 1985, no. 86–1464.
8. Rango N: The social epidemiology of accidental hypothermia among the aged. *Gerontologist* 25(4):424–430, 1985.
9. Johnston JB: Hypothermia: assessment and intervention. *Emerg Nurs Rep* 3(8): 1–7, 1988.
10. Bessen HA: Hypothermia and frostbite. Lecture presented at Scientific Assembly, Atlanta GA, October 25, 1983.
11. Harnett RM, Pruitt, JR, Sias FR: A review of the literature concerning resus-

citation from hypothermia. Part II: selected rewarming protocols. *Aviat Space Environ Med* 54(6):487–495, 1983.

12. Zell SC, Kurtz KJ: Severe exposure hypothermia: a resuscitation protocol. *Ann Emerg Med* 14(4):339–345, 1985.

13. Bangs CC: Hypothermia and frostbite. *Emerg Med Clin North Am* 2(3):475–487, 1984.

14. Ralley FE, Ramsey JG, Wynands JE, et al: Effect of heated humidified gases on temperature drop after cardiopulmonary bypass. *Anesthesia Anal* 63:1106–1110, 1984.

15. Fergusson NV: Urban hypothermia. *Anaesthesia* 40:651–654, 1985.

16. Danzl DF, Sowers MB, Vicaro SJ, et al: Chemical ventricular defibrillation in severe accidental hypothermia. *Ann Emerg Med* 11(12):87–88, 1982.

17. Webb P: Afterdrop of body temperature during rewarming: an alternative explanation. *Amer Physiol Soc* 385–390, 1986.

5.5 ANAPHYLAXIS: A BEE STING

Cathy Robey-Williams, RN, MS, CCRN

Valerie is a 20-year-old white female who was stung on her right hand by a bee, probably a yellow jacket, 30 min ago. She noticed immediate swelling of her hand and arm similar to a reaction which she had with a previous sting. This time, however, she felt different, and she describes the sensation as "edgy all over." When Valerie began feeling a "lump" in her throat and started having difficulty breathing, she called 911.

The paramedic unit found Valerie sitting upright, leaning forward, in obvious respiratory distress. She was edematous, and her color was acrocyanotic. When answering questions, Valerie could only respond in single-word answers. The paramedic applied oxygen at 10 liters/min via a non-rebreather mask. There was very little air movement when her breath sounds were auscultated. Vital signs were BP 80/40, HR 120, and respirations 40. The ECG monitor revealed sinus tachycardia without ectopy. An intravenous line was attempted but was unsuccessful. The ED was consulted, and the paramedic requested the following: epinephrine 0.3 mg, 1:1000 subcutaneous; military antishock trousers (MAST). The physician agreed with the paramedic's request for treatment. The estimated time of arrival was 15 min. Following treatment by the paramedic, Valerie's respiratory status improved. Her BP was 100/50 with the legs of the MAST inflated. During transport a second intravenous access attempt was successful, and Ringer's lactate solution was infused wide open.

On arrival to the ED, Valerie is talking in sentences and states her breathing is much better. She can still feel "that lump" in her throat. Her color is flushed and her skin warm. Valerie's right hand and arm, face, and periorbital area are very edematous. Wheezes are heard in all her lung fields.

Triage Assessment, Acuity Level IV: Severe respiratory distress, respiratory rate 40, acute wheezing, BP < 90 mm Hg.

Valerie is taken immediately to the treatment area where she is kept on oxygen via a non-rebreather mask, and a second liter of Ringer's lactate is hung. Repeat vital signs are BP 100/50, HR 134, and respirations 32. During the interview, Val-

erie tells the emergency nurse that she has no medical history, is not aware of any allergies, and is only taking oral contraceptives. She states she weighs approximately 130 pounds.

Valerie is given a nebulizer treatment with 0.6 mg Alupent in 3 ml NS. The physician orders include 295 mg intravenous aminophylline over 30 min followed by an infusion of 30 mg/hr; 200 mg intravenous Solu-Cortef; and 25 mg intravenous Benadryl. ABG and admission blood work and chest x-ray are also ordered. Following fluid replacement Valerie's BP stabilizes at 110/60, and MAST trousers are reduced. One hour after arrival Valerie appears to be resting comfortably with improvement in her vital signs and breath sounds. Plans have been made for Valerie to be admitted to the hospital for observation overnight.

QUESTIONS AND ANSWERS

1. **What does the term anaphylaxis mean?**

   Anaphylaxis is a Greek term meaning backward protection. The word originates from the early 1900s when Portier and Richet described the responses of dogs to sea anemone toxin. Instead of protecting dogs from the toxin as proposed, repeated exposures to toxin resulted in a hypersensitivity reaction producing massive circulatory collapse and death (1).

   Prior exposure to an antigen is required for anaphylaxis to occur. The antigen is necessary to stimulate IgE antibody formation. The term anaphylaxis can be used broadly to describe any IgE-mediated reaction releasing histamine and affecting target organs which are blood vessels and smooth muscle (2). Most clinicians reserve the term anaphylaxis for severe systemic responses where there is circulatory collapse (2).

   Bee or Hymenoptera stings and penicillin are the two major causes of anaphylaxis in humans (3). The Hymenoptera family consists of honey bees, yellow jackets, wasps, hornets, and fire ants. Hymenoptera venom, a protein, is the antigen that stimulates the chain of events leading to anaphylaxis which accounts for a reported average of 40 deaths per year in the United States (4).

2. **What are the physiological processes that occur during anaphylaxis?**

   There are three separate events that produce anaphylaxis following exposure to a foreign substance: (1) antigen-antibody reaction or complement activation, (2) release of pharmacologically active mediators, and (3) the response of the individual. The initial exposure to an antigen, i.e., the first bee sting, sensitizes a group of B lymphocytes. Plasma cells are then produced which secrete IgE antibodies. The IgE molecule then attaches to the surface of mast cells and basophils (5).

   Subsequent exposures to the antigen produce the chain reaction seen in anaphylaxis. As the antigen enters the body, it attaches to the

IgE molecules that are affixed to the mast cell surface. This added bond activates degranulation of the mast cells and basophils resulting in exocytosis of cell contents. Mast cell exocytosis releases a complex of histamine and heparin which dissociates and circulates into the blood stream. Heparin produces prolonged clotting time. Histamine produces arteriole, venule, and capillary dilatation (3, 5).

There are two types of histamine receptors throughout the body. Stimulation of H1 receptors by circulating histamine results in nonvascular smooth muscle contraction. H2 receptors, when activated, increase gastric secretion which may produce vomiting as well as stimulate cardiac function, which on rare occasions results in ischemic changes on ECG (6). Table 5.5.1 summarizes types of smooth muscle and symptoms that may result when the muscles are affected by histamine.

Several other chemical mediators are released from mast cells and basophils during anaphylaxis: serotonin, kinins, prostaglandins, and leukotrienes. The actions of these mediators combined, contributes to the major respiratory and cardiovascular changes seen with anaphylaxis.

The response of the individual or clinical presentation of anaphylaxis is extremely variable. Symptoms may be mild to irreversible, resulting in death. Reactions to antigens usually occur within 30 min. Factors contributing to an individual's variable response are dose of antigen, route of administration (injection of bee venom from stinger), and the degree of host responsiveness (3).

3. How is a localized reaction to a bee sting differentiated from anaphylaxis?

The body's normal response to a bee sting is first intense burning throbbing pain at the site of venom injection. A small area of inflammation and erythema then develops. This minimal amount of swell-

Table 5.5.1   Histamine Action on Smooth Muscle with Clinical Symptomatology

Smooth Muscle	Histamine Action	Clinical Symptom
Bronchi	Bronchospasm	Wheezing, stridor, dyspnea
Capillaries	Increased membrane permeability	Decreased vascular volume, pulmonary edema
	Angioedema	Uvula and laryngeal edema, choking sensation, dysphonia, barking, crowing, complete airway obstruction
Intestine	Constriction and stimulation of motility	Cramping abdominal pain, vomiting, diarrhea
Bladder	Contraction	Urinary incontinence
Uterus	Contraction	Vaginal bleeding, premature labor

Adapted from Dickerson M: Anaphylaxis. *Crit Care Nurs Q* 11(1):72, 1988, reprinted with permission of Aspen Publishers, Inc., © June 1988.

ing should only pose a threat if the sting occurred in the pharynx affecting breathing or affects distal circulation such as in a ring-bearing finger (7).

Many individuals experience a hypersensitivity reaction to bee stings and other bites such as spiders, mosquitoes, and horseflies. Hypersensitivity reactions are limited to inflammation and erythema, but can affect a larger local area such as the entire arm if the hand is stung. As long as no systemic symptoms occur, the individual is not experiencing a life-threatening emergency. Systemic symptoms of anaphylaxis include itching, paresthesia distal to sting site, generalized erythema, urticaria, angioedema, dyspnea, wheezing, stridor, vocal changes, feeling of impending doom, abdominal pain, vomiting, diarrhea, urinary incontinence, vaginal bleeding, and tachycardia (7, 8).

Individuals experiencing hypersensitivity reactions should be warned that they may develop systemic reactions with future stings. These people should be taught the signs and symptoms and how to obtain proper medical attention.

4. **What are the pharmacological effects of the medications used to treat Valerie?**

A summary of the drugs used, including dosage, and their action is listed in Table 5.5.2.

TIP: The presence of β-blockade medications may decrease the effectiveness of epinephrine. If a patient does not respond to an initial dose of epinephrine, 1 mg intravenous glucagon followed by an infusion of 1 mg/hr is recommended (1, 9).

Table 5.5.2 Common Medications Used in the Treatment of Anaphylaxis

Medication	Dosage	Action
Epinephrine	0.3–0.5 mg of 1:1000 solution s.c. or i.m.; *or* 1:10,000 solution i.v. Titrate to effect. Used when there is evidence of circulatory collapse	Increases contractility and cardiac bronchodilation, constricts aterioles and increases peripheral vascular resistance
Metaproterenol sulfate (Alupent)	0.6 mg aerosol in 3 ml NS	Bronchodilation
Aminophylline	Loading dose: (5 mg/kg body weight) i.v. over 30 min; infusion: 0.5 mg/kg/hr	Bronchodilation
Hydrocortisone (Solu-Cortef)	200–400 mg every 4–6 hr	Stabilizes capillary membrane
Diphenhydramine hydrochloride (Benadryl)	25–50 mg i.v. or i.m.	Blocks histamine receptors; relieves itching, urticaria; decreases angioedema

5. **What nursing diagnoses are applicable to this situation?**
    Nursing diagnoses related to management of Valerie's airway, breathing, and circulatory collapse are crucial. She also requires instruction on management of future potential problems.

    Diagnosis: Ineffective breathing pattern related to a decrease in effective airway size from bronchoconstriction resulting in hypoventilation

    Desired patient outcome: The patient will experience bronchodilation with decreased wheezing, and breath sounds heard clearly in all lung fields. The patient describes relief in the ability to breathe.

    Diagnosis: Impaired gas exchange related to decreased oxygen delivery from alveolar hypoventilation and accumulation of pulmonary interstitial fluid

    Desired patient outcome: The patient will maintain PaO_2 of 90 to 100 mm Hg, and maintain capillary O_2 saturation above 97%; the patient will have clear breath sounds, respiratory rate of 12 to 24, and pink mucous membranes.

    Diagnosis: Decreased cardiac output related to peripheral vasodilation

    Desired patient outcome: The patient will maintain systolic BP $\geq$ 90 mm Hg, HR $\leq$ 100 beats/min, maintain a Glasgow Coma Score of 15, and urinary output $\geq$ 30 ml/hr.

    Diagnosis: Decreased cardiac output related to fluid shift from vascular compartment into interstitial space because of increased vascular permeability

    Desired patient outcome: The patient will experience a decrease in circumferential size of extremities. The patient will have diminished angioedema as evidenced by return of voice, ability to speak clearly, ability to swallow, and decrease in dyspnea.

    Diagnosis: Pain related to body changes and fluid shifts from the chemical action of kinins on body tissue

    Desired patient outcome: The patient will state that there is relief of pain and itching; the patient will not exhibit behavior cues of discomfort.

    Diagnosis: Anxiety related to sympathetic stimulation from the stress response and catecholamine administration

    Desired patient outcome: The patient will verbalize understanding of feelings and sensations resulting from anaphylaxis and medications. Patient will maintain control over anxiety evidenced by calm tone of voice, lack of repetitive motor movement, appropriate discussion, and questions.

Diagnosis: Knowledge deficit related to anaphylaxis and risk of future antigen exposure; treatment techniques

Desired patient outcome: The patient will describe the sequence of events that will result from another bee sting. The patient will describe activities to avoid to decrease her risk, i.e., walking barefoot outside, picnics in August. The patient will return demonstrate technique of subcutaneous injection describing correct dose of epinephrine to be administered using Ana-Kit prescribed to her at discharge. The patient will describe the appropriate steps she would take if she is again stung by a bee.

6. **What nursing interventions should the emergency nurse initiate in this situation?**

Valerie's triage assessment of level IV communicates to the staff that immediate intervention is required. Nursing interventions for Valerie focus on maintaining an adequate airway and treatment of shock. Because a preliminary report was received from the field, equipment for intubation, fluids for resuscitation, and medications were prepared ahead of Valerie's arrival.

The nurse should begin the assessment with airway patency and ventilation effectiveness. Oxygenation should be assessed via neurological status, ABGs, and oxygen saturation. A pulse oximeter is useful to monitor O_2 saturation. Assessment of circulatory status should follow, including cardiac monitoring and obtaining vital signs. Peripheral circulation assessment should include color, temperature, pulse checks, and capillary refill. Urinary output, the most sensitive indicator of cardiac output, should be monitored as soon as Foley catheterization can be accomplished. In Valerie's case, she responded immediately to treatment, and therefore catheterization was not indicated.

As always, Valerie's nurse should introduce his- or herself and explain the planned procedures. The nurse should prepare the patient for the sensations the patient may feel with each medication and procedure. The nurse encouraged Valerie to verbalize her fears or questions, and repeatedly asked her if she was in pain. Medications are administered as ordered to assist with airway clearance. The nurse should be alert to and request medical orders for additional medications such as Benadryl and acetaminophen that will reduce inflammation and itching and provide better comfort for the patient.

After Valerie was comfortable, the emergency nurse taught her about the process of anaphylaxis. The nurse discussed the actions that should be taken following future bee stings, and that a medic alert bracelet was essential to wear. Valerie could easily describe ways to avoid contact with bees in the future and recited the key rules she should follow for safety.

TIP: The decision to admit Valerie for overnight observation was based on the risk of reoccurrence of symptoms that reportedly affects 20% of patients. Secondary reactions can occur up to 8 hrs following anaphylaxis (10).

Prior to Valerie's transfer to the medical unit, the emergency nurse provided a report to the oncoming nurse and suggested that prior to discharge Valerie be given a prescription for an Ana-Kit as well as be taught the technique for self-administration. Valerie was fortunate that she received immediate appropriate care. She will always have to face the danger of this happening again and will have to adapt her life-style to reduce her risk.

REFERENCES

1. Costa AJ: Anaphylactic shock guidelines for immediate diagnosis and treatment. *Postgrad Med* 83(4):368–373, 1988.
2. Valentine MD, Lichtenstein LM: Anaphylaxis and stinging insect hypersensitivity. *JAMA* 258(20):2881–2885, 1987.
3. Netzel MC: Anaphylaxis: clinical presentation, immunologic mechanisms, and treatment. *J Emerg Med* 4(3):227–236, 1986.
4. Hill J: Emergency: anaphylaxis. *Hosp Med* 23(1):19–37, 1987.
5. Barrett JT: Textbook of immunology. St. Louis: Mosby, 1988.
6. Dickerson M: Anaphylaxis. *Crit Care Nurs Q* 11(1):68–74, 1988.
7. Youlten LJF: Anaphylaxis to bee and wasp stings. *Practitioner* 231(1427): 502–507, 1987.
8. Darowski MJ, Hirshman CA: Adrenaline and anaphylaxis. *Anaesthesia* 43(3):253, 1988.
9. Mulleman RL, Pribble JP, Salomone JA: Blood pressure effects of thyrotropin-releasing hormone and epinephrine in anaphylactic shock. *Ann Emerg Med* 17(4):309–313, 1988.
10. Reisman RE, Osur SL: Allergic reactions following first insect sting exposure. *Ann Allergy* 59(6):429–432, 1987.

CHAPTER 6

Reproductive Health System

Overview

The reproductive health system addresses those body structures and processes that relate to physiological sexual function and reproduction. Case studies selected for this section represent high-risk patient situations that could dramatically alter future reproductive ability for the patient.

CUE WORDS

REPRODUCTION
birth process
fertility and infertility
lactation
menopause
menstruation
pregnancy
pregnancy termination

SEXUAL
impotence
puberty
sex hormones
sex organs
sexual function
rape

RELATED NURSING DIAGNOSES

sexual dysfunction
altered sexuality patterns
ineffective breast-feeding
rape—trauma syndrome
rape—trauma syndrome: compound reaction
rape—trauma syndrome: silent reaction

Department of Emergency Medicine Triage Protocols

Reproductive Health System

Level I	Level II	Level III	Level IV
Intermittent but not current swelling of testicle; no pain		Testicular swelling with pain	Testicular swelling; sudden onset of severe pain
Painless penile discharge; penile rash or lesion; positive STD contact	Penile discharge with moderate pain		
Vaginal discharge; mild or no discomfort; itching	Vaginal discharge with normal menstrual history; VSS	Vaginal discharge with severe abdominal pain; last menses abnormal	
Painful menses	Vaginal bleeding; VSS; no orthostasis	Moderate vaginal bleeding with or without pain; orthostatic changes	Severe abdominal pain with or without severe vaginal bleeding; missed or abnormal menstrual cycle
Requests pregnancy test; no associated symptoms	Same as above with documented or suspected pregnancy	Same as above with documented or suspected pregnancy	Same as above with documented or suspected pregnancy, (all patients with pregnancy-related complaints who are more than 14 weeks pregnant by date of their last normal menses should be escorted to labor and delivery)

153

Genital trauma; no acute distress (NAD); "feels sore"	Genital trauma; swelling hematoma; or laceration	Genital trauma with significant bleeding and/or discomfort
History of foreign body in anus, penis, or vagina; has been removed; mild discomfort	Foreign body in anus, vagina, or penis with moderate discomfort	Foreign body lodged in anus, vagina, or penis with severe discomfort
Sexual abuse more than 24 hr ago	Sexual abuse 4–24 hr ago	Sexual abuse within 4 hr

154

6.1 TESTICULAR TORSION: A YOUNG MAN'S DILEMMA
James Jay Hoelz, RN, MS, CEN

Tommy Miller, 13 years old, presents to the triage desk of the ED at 7:00 PM on Monday evening. Tommy is complaining of right testicular pain that he has had for 2 to 3 hr. The pain developed suddenly this evening. Tommy was playing football in gym class this afternoon but denies genital trauma. Tommy admits to three episodes of nausea with vomiting prior to arrival. He denies urinary symptoms such as burning on urination, urgency, or frequency. He is not sexually active and denies a penile discharge.

Tommy's vital signs are temperature 98°F, pulse 120 and regular, respirations 24, BP 130/90. He is slightly diaphoretic and his color is pale. He appears very uncomfortable. His abdomen is soft and his right testicle is enlarged and tender. Testicular torsion is suspected.

Triage Assessment, Acuity Level IV: Severe pain; sudden onset of testicular pain and swelling.

QUESTIONS AND ANSWERS

1. **What is the physiology associated with testicular torsion? How is it repaired?**

During development, the testis descends into the scrotum and is enveloped by the tunica vaginalis, a double-walled membranous lining. An uncovered area attaches to the scrotal wall and anchors the testicle to the scrotum. In some men, the tunica vaginalis envelops the entire testis and the epididymis. The testicle, therefore, is only anchored to the inner layer of the tunica vaginalis and not to the scrotal wall. This results in an unsecured testicle and a condition known as "bell-clapper" deformity.

When activity twists the testicle, blood supply to the area is compromised and pain occurs. The testis is much more prone to twisting in men with "bell-clapper" deformity. Prolonged twisting of the spermatic cord and blood vessels for more than 4 to 6 hr leads to extended vascular compromise and necrosis (1).

There is an 80% success rate of repair of the twisted cord if surgical intervention occurs prior to necrosis. After 6 hr, the success rate drops dramatically and removal of the testis is likely (2). The surgical procedure is an exploration and orchiopexy. Orchiopexy is often performed bilaterally, as a congenital anomaly may possibly exist on both sides and torsion might occur on the other side at some future point.

2. **How is testicular torsion differentiated from epididymitis?**

Epididymitis is an inflammation of the epididymis, most commonly caused by bacterial infection. Symptoms of epididymitis are similar to those of testicular torsion. Since torsion can lead to necrosis and is a surgical emergency, distinguishing between torsion and epididymitis is of the utmost importance. The most common age for testicular torsion to occur is during puberty, ages 12 to 20. Epididymitis is more common after sexual activity has begun. Patients presenting with torsion often complain of sudden onset of severe pain. Patients with epididymitis complain of prolonged, increasing pain and frequently have accompanying symptoms of dysuria and urethral discharge.

On physical exam, the patient with testicular torsion often has a testis that is in a transverse or horizontal position, while the patient with epididymitis has a testis in a vertical position. Another diagnostic tool is the presence of Prehn's sign. A positive Prehn's sign is present when the testicle is supported and elevated and there is relief of pain. Patients with testicular torsion have a negative Prehn's sign and experience no relief of pain with elevation of the testicle. A positive Prehn's sign often occurs with epididymitis (3).

Patients with epididymitis often have an elevated serum WBC count and urinary examination reveals pyuria or WBC in the urine. These indicators are not usually present with testicular torsion (4). A Doppler study will measure a decreased blood flow in the testicle that is twisted or torqued but will often show an increased blood flow with epididymitis (5).

3. **What are the nursing diagnoses appropriate to this situation?**
   Diagnosis: Pain related to ischemia of the involved testicle
   <u>Desired patient outcome:</u>   The patient will state that there is relief or reduction of pain and does not exhibit nonverbal cues of discomfort.
   Diagnosis: Potential for fluid volume deficit related to fluid loss from vomiting
   <u>Desired patient outcome:</u>   The patient will have no orthostasis; will maintain a systolic BP ≥ 90 mm Hg, HR < 100 beats/min, and urinary output > 30 ml/hr; good skin turgor; and moist mucous membranes. The patient will have relief of nausea and vomiting.
   Diagnosis: Knowledge deficit related to normal testicular physiology, occurrence of torsion, and need for surgery
   <u>Desired patient outcome:</u>   The patient (and family) will be able to verbalize a basic understanding of the anatomy of the male reproductive system and the pathophysiology of testicular torsion. The patient will verbalize a basic understanding of hospitalization and surgery such that he will participate in activities of daily living (ADLs) and normal postoperative activities.
   Diagnosis: Fear related to impending surgery

Desired patient outcome: The patient will gain an understanding of the surgical procedure and will describe his fears; the patient will use effective internal and external coping mechanisms
to manage fear; the patient will state that he is less fearful.

4. What are the appropriate nursing interventions for Tommy's care?

The pain associated with testicular torsion is very often severe. The
nurse should gather information on Tommy's coping mechanisms for
pain and his family's expectations about controlling emotions when pain
occurs. Tommy is 13 years old and will likely try to respond in a manner
that will meet his parents' expectations. These responses will give the
nurse an opportunity to identify verbal and nonverbal cues to determine
if adequate analgesia has occurred. The physician may opt to delay pain
medication until a diagnosis has been reached. The nurse should support Tommy and his parents through this period by offering empathy for
Tommy's pain and by explaining the rationale for withholding pain
medication. Once the diagnosis has been made, Tommy should be medicated as ordered with a strong analgesic, usually Demerol.

TIP: For children, it may be helpful to reinforce that the pain is temporary and will go
away, much like going to the dentist or skinning a knee.

The nurse should monitor Tommy's vomiting and frequently assess
him for signs of dehydration. Tachycardia is often the first clinical
sign, and he may complain of dry mouth and fatigue. An intravenous
line will be ordered and initiated. The nurse should monitor flow, vital signs, and urine output to determine adequate hydration.

Testicular torsion is relatively unknown to the lay population, and
time should be set aside early by the physician and the nurse to explain
the pathophysiology of the condition and the steps that will be taken to
repair it. The nurse should be preparing Tommy and his family for the
likelihood of surgery. An unhurried attitude and adequate time will encourage Tommy and his family to feel comfortable asking questions.

Special consideration should be given to Tommy's stage of development. As an early adolescent, Tommy is developing a sense of self-
concept and is adapting to changes in body image. He is probably extremely sensitive about his "private region" and is self-conscious in
speaking about genitalia. Tommy is also at an age when many young
men have begun to masturbate. Tommy may be feeling guilty that his
actions have somehow caused the torsion. These feelings should be
considered when caring for Tommy, and it may be helpful to spend
some time interviewing Tommy without his parents so that he can feel
comfortable sharing his concerns (6).

Testicular torsion is a surgical emergency. Familiarity with the signs and symptoms of the disease process should ensure that the patient is identified as a high-risk patient at triage so that his care is expeditious. Failure to provide expeditious care could result in a poor patient outcome.

REFERENCES

1. Haynes B, Bessen H, Haynes V: The diagnosis of testicular torsion. *JAMA* 249(18):2522–2527, 1983.
2. Wilson J: The treatment of testicular torsion. *Resident Staff Physician,* 28(5): 71–76, 1982.
3. Vogt L, Miller M, McLeod D: To save a testis. *Emerg Med* 20(13):69–76, 1988.
4. Haynes B: Doppler ultrasound failure in testicular torsion. *Ann Emerg Med* 13(12):1103–1107, 1984.
5. Allen T: Testicular torsion: To avert a tragedy, don't wait for a diagnosis. *Consultant* March, 24(3): 301–305, 1984.
6. Murray R, Zentner J: Nursing assessment and health promotion through the life span. London: Prentice-Hall, 1979.

6.2 PELVIC INFLAMMATORY DISEASE
Laura Ann Kress, RN, BSN

Denise is an 18-year-old white female who presents to the triage desk complaining of severe lower abdominal pain that has lasted for 2 days. Denise describes the pain in the midabdominal area, just below the umbilicus. She denies any vomiting but has felt nauseated and has had a decrease in appetite. She also reports fever and malaise since yesterday. Denise's last menstrual period (LMP) was 1 week prior to this visit and was unusually long. She complains of continued spotting with a foul-smelling, yellowish vaginal discharge. She denies use of any birth-control methods.

Denise is accompanied by her boyfriend of 2 months. She is casually dressed, and the zipper of her jeans is open. She is holding her stomach and rocking in the chair. Her temperature is 102° F, BP 120/78, pulse 110, and respiratory rate 22. Denise is not orthostatic.

Triage Assessment, Acuity Level III: Abdominal pain, temperature > 102° F, moderate pain.

Denise is taken to the treatment area by the triage nurse. The triage nurse reports to the treatment nurse that pelvic inflammatory disease (PID) is suspected.

QUESTIONS AND ANSWERS

1. **What is PID and what are the pathogens?**

    PID is a common complication for women who do not seek treatment after exposure to a sexually transmitted disease (STD). PID is an infectious process affecting the ovaries, pelvic peritoneum, pelvic vascular system, pelvic connective tissue, and most commonly the fallopian tubes. Patients at high risk are those with multiple sexual partners, who use an intrauterine device (IUD) for birth control, or have had recent instrumentation of the cervix (i.e., abortions, C-section deliveries, or cervical curettage).

Since PID can affect only some or all of the pelvic structures, patients present with a wide range of symptoms. Most patients complain of mild to moderate abdominal pain, fever, irregular bleeding, and adnexal tenderness. An increase in pain usually occurs following menses. Other signs and symptoms may include nausea and vomiting, malaise, urinary frequency, and vaginal discharge. During the early stage of the disease the patient is relatively asymptomatic, with no pain and only a moderate discharge. Therefore, early treatment is usually not sought.

The incidence of PID is not known. However, in the United States each year more than 900,000 women are diagnosed with the disease (1). *Nesseriam gonorrhoeae* is an anaerobic, Gram-negative diplococci that causes gonorrhea in both men and women. Although not all PID is caused by *N. gonorrhoeae,* the percentage of those cases due to *N. gonorrhoeae* infection is estimated at 20 to 80% (1).

The second bacteria involved in PID is *Chlamydia trachomatis* and is responsible for between one-fourth and one-half of all cases of PID (1). The incidence of chlamydia infection is estimated at three to five million Americans each year (2). The major threat of both types of infections is that infected individuals are usually asymptomatic and do not receive treatment until pain and complications occur. This may be as late as 3 to 4 weeks after the initial contact, and the individual may have spread the infection to other partners.

TIP: Frequently gonorrhea and chlamydia are present simultaneously. Therefore, while cultures are important for specific diagnosis, it is equally important to treat for both bacterium until the culture results are known.

---

2. **What is the morbidity and mortality of PID?**

Although mortality is rare, the morbidity of the disease can cost the health care system millions of dollars every year. Women diagnosed with PID increase their risk of infertility and ectopic pregnancy due to scarring of the fallopian tubes. One long-term study showed that 25% of all women who had PID were unable to conceive children during the subsequent 10 years (1). Moreover, the risk of having an ectopic pregnancy is 6 to 10 times greater (1). The overall incidence of ectopic pregnancy has increased between 1970 and 1983, accounting for a large number of maternal-related deaths, second only to toxemia (3).

3. **What can Denise expect in the treatment area?**

In the treatment area Denise is placed in a room and prepared for a pelvic exam by the physician. The physician will obtain samples of the discharge to culture for gonorrhea and chlamydia and may also ask for a serological test for syphilis, since more than one disease can occur simultaneously. The physician will also do a bimanual exam to detect any pelvic masses that may suggest an abscess or ectopic pregnancy. This part of the exam may be extremely painful for Denise since any movement of the cervix causes an increase in abdominal pain. This "cervical motion tenderness" is sometimes described as a "classic" sign of PID.

Patients diagnosed with PID may be treated on an outpatient basis. Patients routinely hospitalized are those women with peritoneal signs such as abdominal pain with rebound tenderness, temperature greater than 103°F, and decreased intestinal motility. Patients who have a history of pelvic abscesses or pregnancy and who have demonstrated or who currently demonstrate an inability to follow an outpatient regimen are also candidates for admission. Prompt antibiotic treatment is recommended before cultures are available. There is evidence that infertility follows salpingitis (infection of the fallopian tubes) less frequently when treatment is started within 2 days of the beginning of symptoms (4). Current Centers for Disease Control (CDC) guidelines (5) for outpatient management of patients with PID are listed in Table 6.2.1.

4. **What are the nursing diagnoses appropriate for Denise's problem?**
   Diagnosis: Pain related to inflammation of the cervix, uterus, and fallopian tubes
   Desired patient outcome: The patient will state that there is a relief or a reduction of pain and does not exhibit nonverbal cues of discomfort.
   Diagnosis: Infection related to N. **gonorrhoeae** *or* C. **trachomatis** *located in the pelvic cavity*
   Desired patient outcome: The patient's infection will show evidence of resolution demonstrated by temperature of 98.6 to 99.6°F, skin cool, and reported relief of malaise.
   Diagnosis: Knowledge deficit related to how the disease occurs, drug therapy, and safe sex practices
   Desired patient outcome: The patient and her significant other will be able to verbalize a basic understanding of the transmission of sexually transmitted diseases and safe sex practices. The patient will also verbalize an understanding of the proper way to take her medications, including frequency, length of treatment, and side effects. The patient will describe her plan to receive follow-up therapy.

Table 6.2.1 Recommendations for Outpatient Treatment of PID

Drug	Dose	Patient Education
Cefoxitin	2.0 g i.m.	1. Instructions for taking medicine, including dosage, timing, length of treatment. Patient needs to understand that all medication should be taken, even if symptoms subside.
or		
Amoxicillin	3.0 g oral	
or		
Ampicillin	3.5 g oral	2. Advise patient to return for follow-up for side effects or other difficulty with medication or if symptoms continue or increase in severity.
or		
Aqueous procaine penicillin G with probenecid	4.8 million U i.m. 1.0 g oral	
or		
Ceftriaxone	250 mg i.m.	3. Patients should abstain from sexual activity or, if unable to do so, use of condoms is necessary until treatment is completed.
Followed by		
Doxycycline	100 mg oral b.i.d. × 10–14 days	4. Advise patient to stop sexual activity if similar or other STD symptoms recur and return to clinic for health care.
or		
Tetracycline HCL (contraindicated in pregnancy and less active against certain anaerobes)	500 mg oral q.i.d. × 10 days	5. Encourage use of barrier contraceptive methods, especially condoms, to prevent STDs.
Alternative regimens		
Erythromycin base or stearate	500 mg oral q.i.d. × 7 days	
or		
Erythromycin ethyl succinate	800 mg oral q.i.d. × 7 days	

From Shattuck JC: Pelvic inflammatory disease: Education for maintaining fertility. *Nurs Clin North Am* 23(4):903, 1988. (Adapted originally from CDC Guidelines, August 1985.)

Diagnosis: Potential for fluid volume deficit related to fever, infection, and decrease in appetite

<u>Desired patient outcome:</u>   The patient will remain hydrated with systolic BP > 90 mm Hg, HR < 100 beats/min, and urinary output > 30 ml/hr. The patient will drink 1000 ml of fluid during this visit.

5.   What nursing interventions are required for Denise?

In order for Denise to be treated on an outpatient basis, she will need specific instructions about her treatment and disease process. Denise should be instructed to maintain pelvic rest during her treatment phase. This requires reclining in a semi-Fowler's position with the feet elevated in order to avoid strain on adjacent pelvic structures. The semi-Fowler's position also helps to prevent the infection from spreading upward. The use of acetaminophen for fever and pain control can be prescribed. The importance of maintaining adequate fluid and nutritional intake is also important in the healing process.

Explicit instructions on taking the medications should include dosage, timing, and length of treatment. Denise should have a follow-up exam in 2 to 3 days when the culture results are known and at the completion of her antibiotic course. Denise needs to be instructed to return to the ED if her symptoms have not subsided or become worse in 2 to 3 days.

Denise needs to be educated on safe sex principles. These should include abstinence of intercourse until both she and her boyfriend have completed treatment. Birth-control methods such as condoms and vaginal contraceptive creams and jellies used in combination can be an effective barrier against bacteria, decreasing her risk of recurrent infection. She should be advised to report any suspicious symptoms in order to obtain earlier treatment decreasing the chance for further complications of infertility and chronic pelvic pain.

REFERENCES

1. Horsburg C, Douglas J, LaForce M: Preventive strategies in sexually transmitted diseases for the primary care physician. *JAMA* 257(6):815–821, 1987.

2. McElhose P: The "other" STD's as dangerous as ever. *RN* 51(6):52–59, 1988.

3. Honigman B: Ectopic pregnancy. In: Rosen P (ed). Emergency medicine concepts and clinical practice, 2nd ed. St. Louis: Mosby, 1591–1603, 1988.

4. Dornbrand L, Hoole A, Fletcher R, Pickard C (eds.): Manual of clinical problems in adult ambulatory care. Boston: Little, Brown, 322–324, 1985.

5. Shattuck J: Pelvic inflammatory disease: education for maintaining fertility. *Nurs Clin North Am* 23(4):899–906, 1988.

6.3 ECTOPIC PREGNANCY
Patricia C. Bent, RN, CEN

Denise is a 23-year-old black female who presents to the ED accompanied by her husband. She is complaining of sudden onset of right lower quadrant abdominal pain that woke her from sleep 1 hr prior to arrival. She describes the pain as "knife-like" in nature without radiation. She has nausea, but no vomiting. Her LMP was 6 weeks ago, and her past menstrual period (PMP) was normal. She denies any vaginal bleeding at present, but states that she had some spotting about 1 week ago. She discontinued using an IUD 6 months ago in order to become pregnant with her first child. Her vital signs are pulse 110, BP 60 by palpation, respirations 24.

Triage Assessment, Acuity Level IV: severe abdominal pain with missed menstrual cycle, systolic BP < 90 mm Hg, and increased HR.

Denise is escorted immediately to the treatment area as the triage nurse suspects an ectopic pregnancy. Her repeat vital signs are temperature 36.7° C, pulse 122, respirations 24, BP 54/P. Two large bore peripheral catheters are placed with 0.9% NS infusing at a wide open rate. Blood samples are drawn and sent to the lab for chemistry, hematology, blood bank sample, and β human chorionic gonadotropin (HCG) test. Spun hematocrit is 30%. A room air ABG is obtained, and oxygen at 4 liters nasal cannula is administered. Denise is placed in a modified Trendelenburg position for placement of a right subclavian line with another liter of 0.9% NS run at a wide open rate. After 500 ml of fluid, Denise's BP is 106/60, with an HR of 112. A Foley catheter is inserted with an initial output of less than 50 ml. A consultation with a gynecologist is obtained by the ED physician.

The physical exam repeated by the gynecologist reveals a pale-looking, anxious female with severe abdominal pain. Her lungs are clear. The cardiac monitor shows sinus tachycardia. Her abdomen is slightly distended, very firm with minimal bowel sounds and severe pain and guarding on gentle palpation. Her rectal exam is negative for occult blood. The pelvic exam shows a normal uterus with a right adnexal mass. A culdocentesis is performed with aspiration of nonclotting blood. The serum pregnancy test is reported as positive. The diagnosis is made of a ruptured ectopic pregnancy. The patient is immediately prepared to be taken to the OR for exploration and repair.

QUESTIONS AND ANSWERS

1. What is an ectopic pregnancy?

Implantation of a fertilized ovum at a location other than the uterine cavity is known as an ectopic pregnancy. The implantation may be tubal (most common), abdominal, or ovarian. Any woman of childbearing age is susceptible to an ectopic pregnancy. Clinical characteristics include a mean age of 28 years, prior pregnancies, previous ectopics, and nonwhite women (1). There has been an overall increase in the incidence of ectopic pregnancy between 1970 and 1983 (4.5 to 14.0 ectopic pregnancies per 1000 pregnancies). Death due to ectopic pregnancy is the second leading cause of pregnancy-related deaths, after toxemia. An ectopic pregnancy may result from a number of different causes. These include, but are not limited to, previous intrauterine infections, inflammatory changes such as previous ectopics, IUD usage, tubal ligation, and previous gynecological surgeries (2, 3).

Damage to fallopian tubes from previous episodes of PID is the most common cause of ectopic pregnancy (3). This may be due to incomplete healing and scarring of tubal mucosa, creating a partial tubal obstruction and impediment to the passage of an ovum (4). The risk of ectopic pregnancy in patients who have undergone tubal ligation and subsequently become pregnant is approximately 50% (5). Present or recent past use of an IUD may stop the egg from implanting in the uterine lining, making the fallopian tube a more favorable spot (6). Hormones may impede ovum transport thereby mechanically stopping the forward motion of the egg in the fallopian tube (7).

2. **What are the usual signs and symptoms of an ectopic pregnancy?**

In a majority of cases, slight to moderate vaginal spotting may occur after a missed period. Bleeding occurs when the endocrine support of the endometrium becomes inadequate (8). Nausea and vomiting occur as well as abdominal distention when intraperitoneal bleeding occurs. Cullen's sign (a blue discoloration around the umbilicus) is uncommon, but can be diagnostic of hemoperitoneum. When an ectopic pregnancy occurs or ruptures, pain is present most of the time. The pain may vary in type, location, and duration. The pain may be unilateral or bilateral, continuous or intermittent, sharp or cramping. Excruciating abdominal pain in a young, healthy female strongly suggests a ruptured ectopic pregnancy (9). Cardiovascular changes due to hypovolemia may or may not be present in early rupture. When 10% of the circulating blood volume or approximately two units of blood is lost, objective signs of shock may be noted. Loss of circulating blood volume initiates the chain of physiological reactions (tachycardia, vasoconstriction) that occur with a decrease in cardiac output.

TIP: Brown-skinned persons may appear yellow-brown, while black-skinned individuals appear ashen gray when vasoconstriction occurs as a compensatory mechanism in shock (10).

Tachypnea is a subtle sign to be alert for in situations of ectopic pregnancy. Initially the respiratory rate increases as a result of hormonal stimulation. Pain and anxiety may also contribute to hyperventilation. Later, respiratory compensation may occur to combat the acidosis of shock.

3. **Since the signs and symptoms are very similar to other patient situations, for example, ruptured appendix, what tests are done to differentiate an ectopic pregnancy?**

Routinely, a β-HCG will be drawn to determine the presence of a pregnancy. Levels usually rise within 7 days after ovulation and double every 48 hr.

TIP: β-HCG aids in confirming that a pregnancy exists or did exist over the past 1 to 3 weeks.

If the patient is stable and can tolerate transfer to the radiology department, ultrasound can be useful to confirm or exclude an intrauterine pregnancy. A patient who has a positive β-HCG and positive intrauterine pregnancy is not likely to have an additional ectopic pregnancy. The absence of an intrauterine pregnancy in the presence of a positive β-HCG, increases suspicion of an ectopic pregnancy. Ultrasonography is an ideal diagnostic aide as it is of low risk to the patient and provides significant information. Culdocentesis may be a desirable procedure to use when β-HCG results and ultrasound are not immediately available.

4. **What is a culdocentesis, and what is the nurse's role in assisting the physician with this procedure?**

   The patient is placed in a lithotomy position (knees and hips flexed and heels resting on foot rests) and an unlubricated speculum is inserted. A needle attached to a 20-ml syringe is inserted through the posterior fornix into the cul-de-sac. This area is then aspirated to determine the presence of blood. A culdocentesis is said to be positive if the nonclotting blood is found in the cul-de-sac. The nurse's role includes gathering the necessary instruments, positioning the patient, and offering support throughout the procedure. The nurse can help the patient relax by having her breathe through her mouth and relax her abdominal muscles.

5. **What are the nursing diagnoses of concern for the management of this patient?**

   Nursing diagnoses for this patient are identified by characteristics of hypotension and severe blood loss, significant discomfort, fear related to sudden illness, and knowledge deficit related to the need for surgery. Denise is also losing a pregnancy that she desired.

   Diagnosis: Fluid volume deficit related to ruptured fallopian tube with escape of blood into the abdominal cavity

   Desired patient outcome: The patient will maintain a systolic BP ≥ 90 mm Hg, HR ≤ 100 beats/min, and urinary output ≥ 30 ml/hr; the patient will remain oriented to person, place, and time; skin will remain warm and dry.

   Diagnosis: Pain related to ruptured intrauterine structures causing peritoneal irritation

   Desired patient outcome: The patient will state that there has been a reduction in pain; the patient will appear more comfortable until she is transported to the OR and sedated.

   Diagnosis: Knowledge deficit related to what an ectopic pregnancy is and why surgery is necessary

   Desired patient outcome: The patient will be able to state the reason for surgery, actions, and events that will occur and her role in the recovery process.

>**Diagnosis:** *Fear related to potential complications of the surgical procedure*
>> <u>Desired patient outcome:</u> The patient will verbalize a good understanding of the surgical procedure and will state that she feels less fearful.
>
>**Diagnosis:** *Anticipatory grieving related to loss of pregnancy*
>> <u>Desired patient outcome:</u> The patient will discuss the loss of her pregnancy and, as able, will begin the experience of grieving in a supportive environment.

6. **What are the nursing interventions appropriate to initiate in order to resolve these patient problems?**

As with any patient situation in which there is a decrease in cardiac output, maintaining circulating blood volume and ensuring adequate tissue perfusion is essential. The nurse will routinely assist the physician in establishing two large bore intravenous catheters for rapid volume replacement and blood administration. A central venous pressure (CVP) catheter is usually inserted to serve as a guide for fluid replacement. Rapid infusions are administered until the CVP rises 5 cm H_2O above baseline, or the patient's clinical condition improves. The patient is placed in a desirable supine position by elevating the head with a pillow, and elevating the lower extremities 20 to 30°, keeping the knees straight. Oxygen is administered to augment the oxygen-carrying capacity of arterial blood. Care should be taken not to overheat the patient since unnecessary vasodilatation could occur. A Foley catheter is inserted to monitor urine output. Pain is a difficult problem for a patient with an ectopic pregnancy, since the use of narcotics is not recommended. Other means should be tried to make the patient more comfortable. A quiet soothing tone of voice and careful positioning are nursing actions that may help alleviate some discomfort. Distraction is also helpful particularly if a family member is present and capable of offering emotional support. The patient's knowledge deficit may also be contributing to pain and anxiety. Explain the procedure in simple, concise terms, allowing the patient time to ask questions. The important role of patient participation in postoperative recovery should be included. The patient should be allowed to express her feelings of anger or sadness at the loss of the pregnancy if she desires. Her husband should be included in this process if she identifies him as a source of support for her. She should be encouraged to view her feelings as a normal reaction and part of the grieving process.

After a diagnosis of ruptured ectopic was made, Denise was rapidly transported to the OR. A laparotomy was performed, and 1500 ml of blood was found in her abdominal cavity. The right ovary and fallopian tube were removed. She received four units of blood during the procedure. Her postoperative course was uncomplicated, and she was discharged on the fourth postoperative day.

The role of the emergency nurse in assessment and intervention should not be underestimated, since early recognition of ectopic pregnancy may be the single greatest factor in preventing death, irreversible tubal damage, and complete loss of reproductive ability in a very young woman (11).

REFERENCES

1. Centers for Disease Control (CDC): Ectopic pregnancy in the United States. In: CDC Surveillance Summaries, *MMWR*. 53:29ss–37ss, August 1968a.
2. Honigman B: Ectopic pregnancy. In: Rosen P, Baker FJ, Barken RM, et al., eds.: Emergency medicine: concepts and clinical practice. 2nd ed. St. Louis: Mosby, 1591–1603, 1988.
3. Glebatis DM, Janerich DT: Ectopic pregnancies in upstate New York. *JAMA* 249:1730–1735, 1983.
4. Eschenbach DA: Acute pelvic inflammatory disease. *Urol Clin North Am* 11:65–81, 1984.
5. Weckstein LN, Boucher AR, Tucker H, et al.: Accurate diagnosis of early ectopic pregnancy. *Obstet Gynecol* 65:393–397, 1985a.
6. Cheeseman GS: Patient teaching manual 2. Springhouse, PA: Springhouse, 271, 1987.
7. Olds SB, London ML, Ladewig PA, et al.: Obstetric nursing. Menlo Park, CA: Addison-Wesley, 360–361, 1982.
8. Pritchard JA, Mac Donald PC, eds.: Williams obstetrics. New York: Appleton-Century-Crofts, 16:148, 1985.
9. The nurses reference library. Intermed Communications Diagnostics. Springhouse, PA: Springhouse Corp., 1983.
10. Olds SB, London ML, Ladewig PA, Davidson S: Obstetric nursing. Menlo Park, CA: Addison-Wesley, 563–566, 1982.
11. Johnston JB: Ectopic pregnancy. *Emerg Nurs Reports* 2(12):3, March 1988.

CHAPTER 7

Sensory Health System

Overview

The sensory health system relates to the integrity of the senses including proprioception, taste, smell, hearing, vision, and perception of pain. Alterations in these senses could be mechanical or physiological.

Two cases have been selected to demonstrate an alteration in sensory perception (alteration in vision) with different etiologies but similar patient effect and concern. For most patients presenting to the ED, pain is the impetus for seeking help. Many of the case studies throughout this series have had pain and pain management integrated into the overall care plan for the patient. The severity of pain rating by the patient is a defining characteristic for identifying the patient acuity level in the triage system presented.

CUE WORDS

SENSORY PERCEPTION	PAIN
hearing	acute
proprioception	chronic
smell	ache
taste	pressure
touch	soreness
vision	throbbing

RELATED NURSING DIAGNOSES

pain
chronic pain
altered sensory perception (specify)
unilateral neglect

Department of Emergency Medicine Triage Protocols

Sensory Health System

Level I	Level II	Level III	Level IV
Reddened, itching eyes for several days; no sight loss		Reddened, itchy eyes with periorbital edema	Sudden decrease or loss of vision, severe eye pain
Periorbital edema without trauma or associated symptoms	Foreign body sensation present; no hx of foreign body entry; no foreign body present		Chemical splash in eye(s); foreign body; eye irrigated at scene
Chronic eye pain; gradual vision change			Periorbital swelling; bruising with direct trauma; sudden severe eye pain
Corneal abrasion more than 24 hr ago	Corneal abrasion within 24 hr	Corneal ulcer	Penetrating trauma to eye
	Cold injury to external ear		Amputation of external ear
Nonbloody ear drainage; temperature < 102°F	Nonbloody ear drainage; temperature > 102°F	Bloody drainage from ear; no hx of trauma	Bloody drainage from ear after trauma
Gradual hearing loss; no history of trauma	Gradual hearing loss with history of trauma	Acute onset of hearing loss	
Foreign body in ear; no discomfort	Foreign body in ear; complains of mild pain		Foreign body in ear with severe pain; bug in ear

Tinnitus with temperature > 102°F

Tinnitus; hx of aspirin ingestion or vertigo

Incapacitating pain

Mild to moderate pain; periodic or intermittent

Moderate to severe pain; persistent

170

7.1 LOSS OF VISION: ACUTE ANGLE-CLOSURE GLAUCOMA

Leticia V. M. Nanda, RN, MS

Anne is a 60-year-old, slightly obese, white female who is brought to the ED by her husband at 2 o'clock in the morning. She has been experiencing severe, deep, boring pain; decreased vision acuity; and redness and photophobia of her left eye (OS) for the last 7 to 8 hr. A private physician had seen her earlier when she was having mild to moderate ocular complaints, and she was diagnosed with having viral conjunctivitis. She was advised to apply cool compresses to OS and take Tylenol two tablets every 4 hr for eye pain. Over the next few hours her OS pain has rapidly increased in intensity and her vision has become worse.

Triage Assessment, Acuity Level IV: sudden decrease in vision, severe eye pain.

In the treatment area, Anne reports that she has had four similar episodes of ocular problems in the last 5 weeks but that her vision had improved and the pain had disappeared spontaneously after 1 to 2 hr.

Anne is alert and oriented x3, and her skin is warm and dry. Her respirations are deep and regular. Peripheral pulses are strong and regular.

Anne reports having a fairly active life-style and denies any medical problems except a history of upper respiratory tract infection 2 to 3 weeks ago, which has completely resolved. She states she has been very upset over the death of her only daughter from an automobile accident 2 weeks ago.

The physician's ocular findings are reported as follows: Right eye (OD) vision 20/20, OS vision 20/100 PHNI (no improvement over pinhole). OD shows a shallow anterior chamber (AC) and narrow angle, otherwise within normal limits. OS shows a 5- to 6-mm dilated and nonreactive pupil. Extraocular movements (EOMs) are full, and external exam is normal. The left eye slitlamp exam (SLE) shows the conjunctiva 2+ injected; the cornea has moderate stromal edema; the AC is shallow, with trace cells or flare; the iris is very convex; lens is clear. Funduscopic exam of the left eye reveals poor view of the fundus. Tension by applanation tonometer shows the right eye at 12 mm Hg and the left eye at 60 mm Hg. Gonioscopy of the right eye shows a narrow angle; the left eye angle is closed x360°.

The medical diagnosis is acute angle-closure glaucoma of the left eye.

QUESTIONS AND ANSWERS

1. **What is the pathophysiological basis for Anne's ocular problem?**

   The aqueous humor of the eye is a relatively cell-free, protein-free, transparent fluid produced by epithelial cells of the ciliary body and secreted into the posterior chamber. The aqueous humor flows through the pupil and enters the vascular system of the eye through the corneoscleral trabecular meshwork and canal of Schlemm (1). The intraocular pressure (IOP) reflects the balance between the rate of aqueous fluid formation and the amount of resistance to its outflow from the AC into the venous system. In the normal eye, the IOP is relatively constant with a normal range of 10 to 21 mm Hg. The IOP is increased when there is marked obstruction in aqueous outflow from the AC as seen in most kinds of glaucoma. In very few cases, IOP may be raised by hypersecretion of aqueous fluid or high central venous pressure (2). Elevated IOP will eventually cause damage to the optic nerve if not recognized early and controlled. Patients with IOP greater than 21 mm Hg need further evaluation, because they are at higher risk of developing glaucoma (1,3).

The glaucomas may be subdivided according to their mechanism of development into primary (chronic) open-angle glaucoma, primary angle-closure glaucoma, and the secondary glaucomas. Primary open-angle glaucoma accounts for the majority of all cases of glaucoma. The primary angle-closure glaucomas are diagnosed in a smaller population of glaucoma patients.

In acute angle-closure glaucoma, the primary cause of elevated pressure is closure of the AC angle. There is an apposition of the peripheral iris to the trabecular meshwork blocking the aqueous humor from the outflow facilities. The sudden increase in the IOP as the angle closes rapidly causes dramatic symptoms. The patient has severe eye pain, the pupil becomes nonreactive or slightly reactive to light, vision is blurred or foggy, and the patient sometimes sees colored halos around lights. The patient frequently experiences severe headache and sometimes nausea and vomiting (1,4). The pain that Anne is experiencing is due to the rapid and persistent rise in the eye pressure. Blurred or lost vision and colored halos around lights are attributed to corneal edema from the rapid rise in pressure (1,2). Paralysis of the pupillary sphincter from pressure elevation causes mydriasis (1). Venous congestion is manifested by conjunctival injection, engorgement of iris blood vessels, and, sometimes, central retinal vein occlusion. These occur when the IOP is greater than that of the intraocular veins (1). Autonomic stimulation causes nausea and vomiting. Bradycardia and sweating are also noted as effects of oculocardiac reflex activation during the acute attack of angle-closure glaucoma (1).

2. **What are the predisposing as well as precipitating factors for Anne's ocular problems?**

Acute angle-closure glaucoma is a relatively rare disease which accounts for a small percentage of all causes of glaucoma. The occurrence of acute angle-closure glaucoma is an emergency which demands prompt diagnosis and intervention. An IOP of 50 mm Hg or above may produce irreversible ocular damage within a few hours resulting in significant permanent loss of vision if management is delayed (5).

A patient with a very shallow AC or a very narrow chamber angle, who is hypermetropic, is predisposed to having acute glaucoma (2). The anatomical narrowness of the AC angle is positively correlated with the development of acute glaucoma. Acute glaucoma very rarely occurs before the age of 50 (6). Acute angle-closure glaucoma is more common in women than men (5,7). An interesting finding is that acute glaucoma is not common in the black population even when there is an anatomical narrow chamber angle or a convex iris (2).

In anatomically predisposed eyes, acute glaucoma can be precipitated with the use of mydriatic agents (7). Drugs or any circumstances that cause pupillary dilation such as dim light, sympathetic nervous system stimulation (e.g., strong emotion), and others can precipitate an acute attack. Stronger miotics, particularly cholinesterase inhibitors, are known to precipitate angle-closure glaucoma (1,2).

An accurate history of the patient's acute onset of attack usually points to the diagnosis of acute angle-closure glaucoma, even before the patient is examined. However, there are special tools that can confirm the diagnosis.

3. **What are the special tools used to confirm Anne's medical diagnosis?**

Slitlamp biomicroscopy is an ophthalmic tool utilized to examine the frontal view of the outer part as well as the AC of the eye. The patient and the examiner sit on opposite sides of the slitlamp during the exam.

TIP: The patient must keep his or her forehead firmly against the forehead rest for better examination of the eye and, thereby, a more accurate diagnosis.

Injected conjunctiva, corneal edema, presence of cells or fibrin in the aqueous fluid, and presence of a very shallow AC are some signs of acute glaucoma that can be seen with the slitlamp.

A tonometer is used to measure the IOP. There are two types commonly used: the Schiötz and applanation tonometers. The Schiötz tonometer is the more traditional instrument. It is relatively inexpensive and more widely used. However, it can be unreliable, especially in severe myopia, and frequently can cause corneal abrasions. The applanation tonometer is safer and more accurate than the Schiötz but is more expensive. The Schiötz tonometer is held on the patient's cornea while the patient is in a lying position. Topical anesthesia is applied on the cornea before the procedure. The extent to which the plunger of the tonometer indents the cornea is shown on a scale. A conversion table is used to convert the scale reading to the corresponding intraocular pressure. During acute glaucoma, IOP may be 40 to 100 mm Hg.

The gonioscope is a tool used to look at the AC angle and search for the cause of aqueous obstruction in glaucoma. Gonioscopic lenses may be indirect wherein the angle being examined is reflected through a mirror, or the angle can be examined directly. During acute glaucoma, extensive closure of the angle will be found. The presence of peripheral anterior synechiae may be detected through the use of a Zeiss four-mirror lens with the slitlamp microscope.

4. **What are the current medical interventions used to treat Anne's problems and the nursing implications in the use of these measures?**

Once the diagnosis of acute angle-closure glaucoma is established, medical treatment is initiated as soon as possible. The nurse should anticipate the physician to order pressure-lowering agents for the eye, such as pilocarpine 2 to 4%, 1 or 2 drops instilled on the affected eye at frequent intervals; Timoptic 0.25 to 0.5% or equivalent; oral glycerol 50% 0.7 to 1.5 ml/kg body weight; and 250 to 500 mg oral or intravenous Diamox. Intravenous mannitol 20% 1 to 2 gm/kg body weight may be ordered if the above eye medications fail to lower the IOP. Analgesics such as Tylenol, Demerol, or morphine are also needed to relieve the pain. Demerol injection is usually preferred because it is not likely to produce nausea and subsequently vomiting. The IOP is expected to decrease within a few minutes after administration of medications. If the IOP is refractory to intensive medical treatment, the patient should undergo surgical intervention without further delay (2). Otherwise, extensive damage to the optic nerve with permanent loss of vision will occur. Peripheral iridectomy is usually the procedure of choice. With technological advancements, laser iridectomy has replaced surgical iridectomy.

The nurse should monitor the patient for ocular as well as systemic side effects of medications. Pilocarpine, a miotic drug, is a parasympathetic agent. The most common side effects are headache, ocular pain, blurred vision, nausea, vomiting, and abdominal pain. Systemic effects are rare and usually occur with very frequent instillations of the drug (8). Timoptic is a β-adrenergic blocking agent. It is contraindicated in patients with asthma, COPD, and heart failure. Orthostatic hypotension can occur. The patient's heart rate should be monitored and Timoptic should be held for bradycardia with physician notification.

TIP: Finger pressure should be applied over the puncta for about 15 to 30 seconds after the eye drops are administered to minimize the risk of system absorption and reaction.

Side effects of hyperosmotic agents such as glycerol and mannitol are headache, nausea, and vomiting. Patients should be monitored for fluid and electrolyte imbalance, dehydration, and fluid overload especially when the patient is on mannitol therapy.

TIP: Strict intake and output measurement is the best way to monitor fluid balance. To minimize nausea and vomiting with glycerol administration, the drug should be mixed with fruit juice over cracked ice and sipped through a straw.

Side effects related to carbonic anhydrase inhibitors such as Diamox are paresthesia, loss of appetite, nausea, vomiting, drowsiness, renal calculi, hypokalemia, fatigue, and depression. The patient's electrolyte balance should be monitored. Diamox should be used cautiously in patients with known allergy to sulfa drugs.

5. **What nursing diagnoses are of high priority in the care of this patient?**
A patient who is suffering from an attack of acute angle-closure glaucoma has similar nursing problems as many patients who have other kinds of ocular emergencies such as alkaline or chemical injuries to the eye, and penetrating injuries (e.g., from a fish hook).

*Diagnosis: **Pain related to increased intraocular pressure***
Desired patient outcome: The patient will state that the pain is relieved or diminished; the patient will not demonstrate nonverbal cues of pain.

*Diagnosis: **Visual sensory-perceptual alteration related to decreased sight and proprioception with visual changes in left eye***
Desired patient outcome: The patient will describe increased visual acuity and ability to place objects in relationship to each other.

*Diagnosis: **Potential for injury related to impaired vision***
Desired patient outcome: The patient will remain free from injury; the patient will demonstrate ways to move and interact with the environment that minimize risk.

*Diagnosis: **Impaired mobility related to impaired vision***
Desired patient outcome: The patient will demonstrate modified behaviors and actions that will allow her to participate in her care.

*Diagnosis: **Anxiety related to pain, sudden diminished vision, unfamiliar environment and procedures***
Desired patient outcome: The patient will describe her feelings of anxiety and use effective coping mechanisms to manage self. The patient will describe an increase in psychological and physiological comfort.

Diagnosis: Knowledge deficit related to acute angle-closure glaucoma, diagnostic procedures, and treatment

Desired patient outcome: The patient will verbalize basic understanding of the disease process. The patient will follow instructions during diagnostic procedures. The patient will participate in the administration of medications and will state the potential side effects that should be reported to the nurse immediately. At discharge, the patient will be able to demonstrate the procedure for administering her own eye drops.

Diagnosis: Potential for ineffective coping related to potential loss of vision

Desired patient outcome: The patient will demonstrate internal coping strategies by asking appropriate questions, seeking assistance from her husband and the nursing staff as required, and participating actively in her care as needed.

Diagnosis: Potential for dysfunctional grieving related to recent death of only child in a traumatic accident

Desired patient outcome: The patient will be able to discuss the recent traumatic event. The patient will state that feelings of loss, alterations in sleep-wake patterns, alterations in desire for food and fluids, lack of interest in outside activities, and so on, are normal responses to the death of a loved one. The patient will be able to identify internal and external supports that can assist her during the grief period.

6. **What nursing interventions are appropriate for Anne based on her diagnoses?**

Having an acute onset of pain and loss of vision can be a very difficult experience for Anne. Anxiety is a prominent feature in any person who comes to the ED with vision changes. A care plan that emphasizes education and the patient's understanding of the disease process, diagnostic tests, and treatments will definitely benefit her.

Besides assessing for the intensity and character of ocular pain, giving ordered analgesics, and evaluating the patient's response, an attentive and caring attitude from the nurse is imperative. Assure the patient that appropriate measures are being implemented. Interdependent nursing actions of prompt administration of medications to lower IOP and monitoring of the patient for complications are indicated. The patient's environment should be controlled to minimize risk of injury. The patient should be placed on a stretcher with side rails up, in a well-lighted room. The call bell should be within the patient's reach. Hazards on the floor between the bed, bathroom, and door should be removed. Anne should be encouraged to ask for assistance with getting out of bed until she is able to demonstrate that she is able to negotiate in her environment.

Teaching should be ongoing, particularly in the use of her medications and their complications. Anne should be asked to participate as she is able in her care.

Anne should be encouraged to grieve for her daughter's death. A social worker may be helpful to Anne and her family in this process. Anne's acute glaucoma may have been precipitated by her emotional response to her daughter's death.

If the patient is admitted to the hospital for further treatment, the nursing report should include Anne's current response to interventions, coping strategies, and understanding of her condition.

REFERENCES

1. Kolker AE, Hetherington Jr J: Becker-Shaffer's diagnosis and therapy of the glaucomas. St. Louis: Mosby, 1983.
2. Chandler P, Grant WM: Glaucoma. Philadelphia: Lea and Febiger, 1979.
3. Hoskins HD, Jr: Definition, classification, and management of the glaucoma suspect. Symposium on Glaucoma. Transactions of the New Orleans Academy of Ophthalmology. St. Louis: Mosby, 1981:19–29.
4. Sheehy SB, Barber J: Emergency nursing, principles and practice. St. Louis: Mosby, 1985.
5. Clark CV, Mapstone R: Diurnal varia-
tion in onset of acute close-angle glaucoma. *Br Med J* April 26, 1986;292:1106.
6. Strong N: Ocular emergencies. *Practitioner* February 22, 1988:232:174–178.
7. Brooks AMV, West R, Gillies WE: The risks of precipitating acute angle-closure glaucoma with the clinical use of mydriatic agents. *Med J Aust* July 7, 1986; 145:34–36.
8. McEvory GK, ed.: American hospital formulary service drug information. Bethesda, MD.:Published by authority of the Board of Directors of the American Society of Hospital Pharmacists. 1989.

7.2 LOSS OF VISION: PENETRATING EYE INJURY

Patricia C. Epifanio, RN, MS, CEN

Mr. J. Jones presents to the triage desk of the ED complaining of a "teardrop" on his right eye. Mr. Jones reports that he had been hammering on a screwdriver in his home workshop yesterday. He was attempting to straighten the screwdriver with a hammer when he felt something fly into his right eye. He suspects it was a metal sliver from the screwdriver. Initially he had a small amount of pain and tearing of his right eye, both of which subsided quickly. It was not until the next day that he realized that he had a teardrop-like protrusion which he describes as being located at the lower margin of the iris and the sclera of his right eye. Mr. Jones does not wear corrective lenses. He was not wearing protective glasses at the time of the injury.

Mr. Jones' primary and secondary assessments are within normal limits. He denies any significant medical problems. He denies smoking and does not use alcohol or recreational drugs. He is on no medications and denies any known drug allergies.

His last tetanus immunization was 2 years ago when he accidently punctured his foot with a nail.

Triage Assessment, Acuity Level IV: penetrating trauma to eye, foreign-body sensation present.

Mr. Jones had bilateral eye patches placed and was taken immediately to the treatment area.

QUESTIONS AND ANSWERS

1. Why is Mr. Jones' case such an acute emergency since he is not experiencing pain and the event occurred yesterday?

Even though Mr. Jones is not experiencing pain, foreign bodies in and around the eye are usually quite painful and can cause significant visual loss if not treated properly. Potential areas for injury are the skin of the eyelid; penetration into the conjunctiva; penetration into the cornea, either superficially or deeply; or deep penetration into the anterior or posterior chambers. Foreign-body injuries to the eye usually occur from shattered particles in work-related accidents (drilling, sanding) from explosions (gunshot, fireworks), or, in the case of children, from sand or dirt.

Common complaints expressed by patients with foreign-body sensations include pain, itchiness, and a sensation that the object is "moving around in the eye." Actually, the foreign body is usually lodged within the conjunctiva under the upper lid and is not moving; but with each blink of the eyelid a different area of the cornea may be irritated giving the impression of foreign-body movement.

Foreign bodies that are lodged in the cul-de-sacs under the upper and lower lids can usually be removed by careful swabbing of the area with a cotton-tip swab and gentle irrigation with normal saline. Conjunctival foreign bodies that are on the surface of the conjunctiva or have only superficially penetrated the conjunctiva of the eyeball (bulbar conjunctiva) can usually be wiped off with a cotton swab or toothless forcep after anesthetizing the eye. Sometimes conjunctival foreign bodies leave an underlying laceration that could lead to infection. Patients, and especially children, with an underlying laceration should be admitted to the hospital for exploration of the wound under anesthesia.

Corneal foreign bodies are very common and are usually embedded. These are not easily removed, and removal is not possible without anesthetizing the cornea with a topical agent. Sometimes irrigating the cornea with sterile saline, directing the flow toward the foreign body, will dislodge the object. If irrigation is unsuccessful, then the use of a cotton swab or removal by needle may be indicated. This procedure is usually performed by an opthalmologist. If the removal of a foreign body is followed by obvious leakage of fluid or there is shallowing of the anterior chamber of the eye on exam, corneal perforation should be suspected and treated immediately by an ophthalmologist.

Foreign bodies that are made of vegetative substances such as wood frequently cause infection. Metallic foreign bodies, especially those made of iron, cause rust to form in the underlying tissue within only 2 to 4 hr. A metallic foreign body that has been lodged for 6 to 8 hr may have a complete rust ring around it. When this occurs, the foreign body may be easily removed but the rust ring remains. Patients who have rust rings may need these removed surgically by an opthalmologist.

If a metallic foreign body remains embedded for several days before medical assistance is sought, necrosis of underlying tissue may occur. Although this necrosis may ease the removal of the foreign body and the rust ring, there is greater risk for infection and corneal ulceration.

Mr. Jones' situation involves a metal object. The object is deeply embedded in the posterior chamber of the eye and a teardrop-like protrusion has formed. This is considered an intraocular foreign body and constitutes a surgical emergency.

2. **What assessments should be performed in evaluating the severity of the patient's injury? What medical interventions are required for Mr. Jones?**

Visual acuity testing is usually performed using the Snellen chart at 20 ft. A Rosenbaum chart, a hand-held version of the Snellen chart, can be used for nonambulatory patients and is held 14 inches from the eyes. Visual acuity should be checked in both eyes, even when an injury or problem is reported in only one eye. The patient should also be checked with corrective lenses in place for comparison. If the patient's glasses are unavailable, then a pinhole test can be performed. A pinhole is put into a 3 × 5 card or any other piece of cardboard, and the cardboard is held up to the patient's eye. This simulates the effect gained from corrective lenses. The visual acuity test helps to determine the degree of visual loss that may be present.

The physician should gently palpate the eye and eye socket of a patient with a penetrating injury to the eye. If the globe has ruptured and there has been extravasation of the vitreous humor, the patient may have "soft eye," a palpated sensation of lost density of the eyeball. Examination of the tissue around the eye will help determine if infection has occurred or if there are other penetrated objects undetected by the patient. The physician frequently will examine the eye with the aid of the slitlamp.

The physician will also usually order soft-tissue x-rays and CAT scan of the eye in order to prepare for surgical removal of a deeply embedded foreign object such as that of Mr. Jones.

At CAT scan evaluation, it was determined that Mr. Jones will require surgery on the posterior chamber of the eye to remove the metal sliver and some of the surrounding necrotic vitreous humor. This type of surgery requires the use of fiber optics. If it is determined during surgery that the patient has experienced significant globe disruption, then enucleation of the eye may need to be performed. This is a potentially catastrophic outcome for a patient who is otherwise healthy and is feeling "fine."

3. **What are the usual medical interventions that the nurse can anticipate once a foreign body has been removed, provided surgery is not indicated?**

Superficial wounds or abrasions caused by foreign-body irritations of the conjunctiva or sclera are usually managed conservatively. Foreign-body penetration into the cornea should be managed with similar considerations as a corneal abrasion. Topical anesthetics for pain should not be used because the cornea will heal too slowly with these applied. If pain relief is needed, then a long-acting cycloplegic such as 1/4% Isopto Hyoscine (scopolamine) is usually ordered and can be instilled. Pain usually occurs from spasm of the cilia, which is a reflex reaction to stimulation of corneal nerve endings. Cycloplegics paralyze the ciliary body muscle, relieving the spasm. If cycloplegics are not indicated, then a systemic nonsteroidal antiinflammatory agent such as acetaminophen can be used.

Infection is a serious consideration when foreign bodies penetrate the cornea. Antibiotic coverage is frequently indicated. If no haze is present on exam around the site of the foreign body, a pressure bandage over the eye after instillation of the antibiotic is indicated for 24 hr.

After 24 hr, the bandage is removed and antibiotics instilled every 3 to 4 waking hours until the epithelium is healed. The pressure patch should not be applied if there is indication of an infection, such as haze in the surrounding tissue. Topical steroids are also avoided as they inhibit wound healing, encourage fungal infections, and in some patients can increase intraocular pressure.

4. **What are the pertinent nursing diagnoses for a patient with an intraocular foreign body?**

Nursing diagnoses for the patient with a penetrating eye injury include the following:

Diagnosis: Pain related to irritation of tissue by foreign object

Desired patient outcome: The patient will state that there is relief of pain or reduction in the sensation of pain to a tolerable level; the patient will not exhibit nonverbal cues of pain.

Diagnosis: Visual sensory-perceptual alteration related to foreign body lodged in visual field and irritation of surrounding tissue; temporary blindness with both eyes patched

Desired patient outcome: The patient demonstrates the ability to adapt and compensate for visual field deficit by maximizing use of his other unimpaired senses.

Diagnosis: Anxiety related to sudden loss of vision and implications of need for hospitalization and surgery

Desired patient outcome: The patient will describe his feelings of anxiety and use effective coping mechanisms to manage self; the patient will describe an increase in psychological and physiological comfort.

Diagnosis: Knowledge deficit related to the medical treatment of intraocular foreign body and home care requirements following surgery

Desired patient outcome: The patient will describe in basic terms the surgical procedure to be performed and implications for recovery; the patient will describe the role he will play in his postoperative care including use of eye drops and dressing changes.

Diagnosis: Potential for injury related to diminished (obstruction) visual field

Desired patient outcome: The patient will remain free from injury; the patient will demonstrate ways to move and interact within the environment that minimize risk.

Diagnosis: Impaired mobility related to impaired vision

Desired patient outcome: The patient will actively participate in his care; the patient will demonstrate modified behaviors and actions that will allow him to participate in his care.

5. **Since Mr. Jones will be admitted for surgery, what nursing actions are appropriate related to these diagnoses?**

Mr. Jones had both eyes patched at triage to reduce ocular movement to prevent further damage or irritation by the metal sliver.

TIP: Because eyes move together, both eyes should be patched even in the presence of single-eye injuries. In cases of a ruptured globe, pressure can be avoided when patching the eyes by using a metal shield or simple paper cup lightly taped over the eye. The areas of pressure should be on the bony orbit. When taping a patch in place, use five 5-inch strips of 1-inch tape. The strips should be placed on the diagonal from the medial orbital rim to the lateral cheek bone so as not to pull on the face. To avoid skin irritation use paper or plastic tape.

Mr. Jones should be placed on a stretcher with side rails up. He should have his call bell within reach. He should be placed in an area of the department where he would feel that he has not been left entirely alone. Sudden blindness, even if only temporary, can be confusing and contribute to alterations in other senses such as hearing and sense of space and time. Having a family member sit with the patient will provide security and reassurance during this period of temporary blindness.

The nurse should be aware of the patient's pain and anxiety and administer medications as indicated. Frequent verbal interactions with offers of reassurance or providing education are helpful. The patient should be informed of normal pre- and postoperative events that will occur and how he will be expected to participate. Questions regarding temporary or permanent loss of sight should be answered honestly, with reassurances that the care being provided will hopefully minimize any permanent problems. The patient should be prepared for surgery in the usual manner. Tetanus diphtheria toxoid or plain tetanus toxoid should be given, if the patient's immunization is not up to date.

At the time of discharge the nursing plan of care should include patient education on strategies to prevent future injury. Mr. Jones should be instructed to wear shatterproof eyeglasses with side shields or protective goggles whether he is at work or at home.

SUGGESTED READINGS

Lubeck, D: Penetrating ocular injuries. *Emerg Med Clin North Am* 1988;6(1): 127–140.

Melamed M: The injured eye at first sight. *Emerg Med* October 15, 1988:86–98.

Nurse's Reference Library: Emergencies. Springhouse, PA: Springhouse, 1985.

Rea R, Bourg P, Parker JG, Rushing D, eds.: Emergency nursing core curriculum. 3rd ed. Philadelphia: Saunders, 1987:485–487, 493–494.

Rosen P, Baker II F, Braen R, Dailey R, Levy R, eds.: Emergency medicine: concepts and clinical practice. 2nd ed. St. Louis: Mosby, 1988:648–649.

Sheehy SB, Barber J: Emergency nursing principles and practice. 2nd ed. St. Louis: Mosby, 1987.

Stokes HR: Ocular foreign bodies. In: Donabred L, Hoole AJ, Fletcher RH, Pichard Jr CG, eds. Manual of clinical problems in adult ambulatory care. Boston: Little, Brown, 1985:19–21.

CHAPTER 8
Social Health System

Overview

An individual's interpersonal relationship with family and community that determines use of resources and services in the maintenance of health are addressed in the social health system. Individuals are dependent on social support and interaction regardless of health status. Individuals who have chronic debilitating illness, who are very young or very old, or who have diminished cognitive abilities have a greater need for help from significant others including family, friends, social workers, social agencies, and community care facilities. Not all individuals are fortunate to receive positive, supportive care for any number of reasons. Limits may include the financial, intellectual, and emotional abilities of the support persons. ED nursing personnel frequently see patients who require a social work referral in order to sort out the complexities of matching care needs to resources available. Sometimes, because of inadequate coping styles and social supports, a patient presents to the ED with clinical signs and symptoms that are the result of abuse or neglect. The ED nurse should be aware of this potential and always assess the patient's social health system along with his or her biophysical health status. Case studies in this section are presentations of abuse that may occur with a child or an elder. The astute ED nurse will not limit his or her concerns to these two categories of patients. Middle-aged persons (male and female) often suffer from abuse and/or neglect and may be even more reluctant to share their social situation with health care workers because of shame over perceived lack of control or poor self-esteem.

For some patients extreme loneliness through chosen social isolation may be a cofactor in health status changes that prompt the need for medical care. This may be the result of a dysfunctional individual or family process.

CUE WORDS

FAMILY	COMMUNITY
abuse and neglect	culture
coping	religion
family planning	services
finances	sexual relations
home maintenance	social interaction
parenting	social isolation
process	

183

RELATED NURSING DIAGNOSES ▬▬▬▬▬▬▬▬

impaired social interaction
social isolation
altered role performance
altered parenting
altered family processes
parental role conflict
ineffective individual coping
impaired adjustment
defensive coping
ineffective family coping: disabling
ineffective family coping: compromised
family coping: potential for growth
diversional activity deficit

Department of Emergency Medicine Triage Protocols

Social Health System

Level I	Level II	Level III	Level IV
Referrals to social work:			
Inadvertently left in hospital without transportation			
Needs transportation to referral center; does not meet criteria for ambulance transport and has no funds			
Presenting for care because prolonged disease disability has exhausted supportive abilities of significant others			
	Removed from unacceptable home environment, i.e., condemned building; needs medical evaluation and social work referral		
Appears to have been abused or PMH has high index of suspicion, or significant other appears to have abuse potential; client is receptive to counseling, will accept social work referral	Presents with injury secondary to abuse or neglect; plans to return to same environment; denies possible recurrence; does not accept psychodynamics	Sustained significant injury secondary to abuse; repeated episodes of abuse and return without counseling; or PMH of increasingly serious abuse or neglect	

8.1 CHILD ABUSE: A BETRAYAL OF THE YOUNG
Laurel Ann Ault, RN, BS

Maurice is a 27-month-old black male brought to the emergency room at 1:50 PM by his mother and maternal grandmother. Maurice's mother states that Maurice has had the chickenpox for 4 days and a temperature, vomiting, and diarrhea since this morning. She further states that Maurice was well when she left for work this morning, leaving him in the care of her boyfriend. However, she was called home by her boyfriend when Maurice "suddenly became ill." Maurice has had no fever medication today.

On initial examination, Maurice is withdrawn and talking in monosyllables. He is lethargic, gray in color, with skin that is hot, dry, and of poor turgor. He is unable to stand, sit up, or hold his head up without assistance. His vital signs are rectal temperature T-103.4° F, pulse-128, respirations-28, and BP 60 by palpation.

Triage Assessment, Acuity Level IV: BP < 90 mm Hg systolic, temperature > 102° F, lethargic.

Maurice is immediately placed in a treatment room. While being undressed, he is noted to have calamine lotion covering his entire body, even where there are no apparent pox lesions. Discolorations of the skin are also apparent under the calamine lotion.

An intravenous line of 5% dextrose and 20% normal saline is established, and bloods are drawn for a CBC with differential, SMA 7, amylase, bilirubin, ammonia level, and blood cultures. He is placed on O_2 by cannula at 3 liters. A stool culture is obtained, and he is bagged for a urine specimen.

Further examination of Maurice, after initial emergency intervention and with the calamine lotion removed, reveals multiple ecchymotic lesions on his chest, abdomen, back, arms, buttocks, thighs, head, and neck. The ecchymotic areas vary in color ranging from red to darker red, to purple, yellow, and green. These lesions are noted to be linear and linear-looped in shape. There is also a healing linear-looped laceration to the upper left posterior thigh with redness and swelling of this thigh. The lesions vary in size from 1.2 × 1 cm to 1.5 × 8.5 cm.

On further interviewing as to the nature and possible cause of the lesions, Maurice's mother first stated she "didn't know" or notice any bruising, and then stated, "Maybe it's because he likes to crawl under the bed." His mother did state that she does slap Maurice occasionally with an open hand, "but he has his clothes on."

Maurice's grandmother stated she has seen Maurice being hit with a belt by his mother. She also stated that she visits everyday to "check on" Maurice. She last saw him yesterday but denies seeing any bruises.

Maurice's mother denies ever seeing her boyfriend strike Maurice. She also states that the boyfriend told her that the bruise on Maurice's head occurred this morning when Maurice pulled a chair up to an unscreened window, climbed on the chair, and leaned out of the window. The boyfriend, fearing Maurice would fall out of the window, ran over, grabbed Maurice, lost his footing, and fell backward, with Maurice hitting his head on the stereo.

Maurice's mother is unmarried. She lives with her boyfriend, Maurice, and a 6-

month-old daughter. Maurice's mother is employed in housekeeping at another hospital. The boyfriend is unemployed and is the father of the 6-month-old daughter, but not of Maurice.

Maurice was admitted to the hospital with the diagnoses of severe dehydration, rule out encephalitis secondary to varicella, gastroenteritis, and suspected child abuse and neglect.

This case study will discuss child abuse and neglect and as such will not address Maurice's medical problems.

TIP: Every child who presents in an emergency room, no matter what the presenting complaint, should be thoroughly examined to rule out possible abuse or neglect. Current statistics on the instances of child abuse are considered minimums as many cases still go unrecognized and/or unreported.

QUESTIONS AND ANSWERS

1. **When evaluating an injured child, what is the most important first and last question to be explored?**

   Is the extent or nature of this injury consistent with the history as given or with the developmental age of the child?

2. **What kinds of wounds, most identifiable with child abuse, are applicable here?**

   The following categories describe current forms of abuse of children. Analysis of the pattern of the injury, as well as repeated injury to a child, are both significant signs for early recognition.

   1. *Bruises and welts.* Studies indicate that bruises and welts are the most common manifestation of child abuse. The primary target zone for these injuries extends from the back of the neck to the back of the thighs. Assessment of bruises of various colors should be noted. Bruising can be dated through color changes: red-blue 1 to 2 weeks, blue-purple 3 to 5 weeks, green 6 to 8 weeks, and yellow-brown 8 to 10 weeks until resolution. If bruises are present and the caretaker(s) deny knowledge of them, inflicting them, or claim the child "bleeds or bruises easily," a bleeding disorder screen (PT, PTT, bleeding time, thrombin time, and platelet count) should be ordered by the physician.

TIP: There should be a high index of suspicion for child abuse when a child presents with bruising in various stages of resolution.

2. *Multiple injuries.* Multiple injuries consist of abrasions, contusions, and lacerations. Other indicators of a repeated pattern of injury to the child are contusions, welts, lacerations, and scar tissue injuries

in multiple stages of healing, such as burns, scratches, lacerations, and bruises of various colors.

3. *Wraparound injuries.* This type of injury is caused by a flexible object such as a belt strap or extension cord. An extension cord leaves marks of a consistent thickness, while belt wounds leave both thin and wide marks in a looping fashion due to the centrifugal force that turns the belt.

4. *Fractures.* Evaluation of all cases of suspected child abuse should include long bone (trauma) x-rays, ordered by the physician. Long bone fractures that are torsion-induced are characterized as spiral fractures of the midshaft or evulsion fractures of the ankle, knee, wrist, or elbow joints. These fractures are usually the result of a twisting motion to the child by an adult. X-rays will also detect any previous untreated fractures, and if detected, will increase the probability that the child has been abused. Any child under the age of 5 in which abuse is suspected should have a trauma survey. Furthermore, a child under the age of 5 with a fracture, or a child with multiple fractures in various stages of healing, particularly under the age of 5, should prompt a high index of suspicion for abuse.

TIP: Bones of children under the age of five are elastic. Extreme force is required to cause fractures.

Maurice presented in the emergency room with multiple injuries, including contusions, a laceration, and bruises in various stages of resolution. The linear-looped lesions appeared to be consistent with wraparound injuries, and the instrument used appeared to be a belt. Child abuse was suspected based on these findings. A bleeding screen was done and showed no abnormality. A long bone (trauma) survey was done and revealed no acute or old fractures.

3. **What is a more subtle indicator of abuse and/or neglect?**

A more subtle indicator of abuse or neglect is evidence of learning disabilities or developmental delays, especially in language and fine motor skills, that cannot be attributed to a specific physical or psychological problem.

A psychological evaluation done 3 days after Maurice was admitted to the hospital revealed socially withdrawn behavior with receptive language skills at the 18 to 20 month level and expressive language skills at the 16 to 18 month level. There was no evidence of autisticlike behavior or pervasive mental retardation. These behaviors are consistent with environmental deprivation.

4. **What is the nurse's role when a diagnosis of inflicted injury is suspected?**

   When a diagnosis of abuse is suspected, the nurse should expedite the evaluation of the child. Cases of suspected child abuse should be given high priority. The reasoning is threefold: (1) There is the potential for the caretaker(s) to elope with the child before intervention can be initiated; (2) consultants may be necessary from other fields and arrangements for them to see the child should be made as quickly as possible; and (3) a child who has already been victimized is at risk of being secondarily victimized when placed in unfamiliar surroundings with unfamiliar people for inordinate amounts of time.

   The nurse should provide pertinent information that will help the physician arrive at the correct diagnosis. In some instances the nurse may consider the diagnosis of child abuse before the physician. If the physician is reluctant to consider the diagnosis or thinks otherwise, the nurse should report it alone.

   Once identified, the nurse should work with the physician to implement protocols on complete medical evaluation of the child. Detailed histories should be obtained from whatever caretaker presents in the emergency room with the child. If the child is old enough, a *brief* history should be obtained from him or her. A lengthy interview may further traumatize the child. On physical exam, detailed notes should include site, shape, size, and color of injuries and whether there is the mark of an identifiable instrument or object.

   If the parent refuses hospitalization for the child or a consultation, the nurse should notify the appropriate law enforcement agency. Each emergency room should have available in the unit a written copy of the law and the hospital's policy and procedure for child abuse patients.

   The nurse should maintain a helping approach toward abusive parents. Feeling angry with abusive parents is natural, but expressing that anger is very damaging to parent cooperation. The nurse should acknowledge that most of these parents are lonely, frustrated, unloved, or otherwise needy people, who actually love their children but who have lashed out at them in anger. The nurse should help the emergency room staff remain supportive and therapeutic in these cases and ensure that the parents are kept informed of what is happening to their child at all times. Stress the emergency room staff's concern for the safety and well-being of their child.

   The nurse should request a child protection team worker consultation. In general, psychosocial evaluations are done by the child protective service social worker. An inside hospital worker such as a social worker or child abuse liaison nurse with expertise in child abuse management should be consulted in all cases of abuse. A child abuse liaison nurse offers not only expertise in emergency medicine, but also in the subtleties of child abuse and neglect through training in this field.

The nurse, physician, or social worker should report suspected child abuse. Most states, by law, require a verbal report within 24 hr, and a written report within 48 hr in all cases of suspected abuse or neglect. This report is not contingent upon a definitive diagnosis of abuse or neglect, only the suspicion of it. This report is made to the local protective services agency. If a health care provider feels the child is in imminent danger of further harm if returned home, or if the caretaker(s) show signs of eloping with the child before the evaluation is completed, an order of shelter care may be obtained from protective services. This order ensures that the child cannot be removed from the hospital or the care of protective services until it is reasonably determined that the child is returning to a safe environment.

The nurse can provide alternative choices for maladaptive parents. Where appropriate, parents can be referred to organizations that provide classes in parenting skills, child growth and development, and stress management. The nurse should be familiar with what programs are available and make appropriate referrals based on this information.

5. **What nursing diagnoses are applicable to this situation?**

The child who is the victim of abuse presents a major challenge to emergency room nurses. The child must be treated for the injuries sustained. The dysfunctional family unit must also be treated. The diagnoses must include not only the child, but the family, to establish optimal and comprehensive care.

Family Diagnoses

Diagnosis: Alteration in health maintenance related to inadequate therapeutic measures in illness or an unhealthy life-style, as evidenced by the delay in seeking medical attention by the caretaker (no fever medication given to the child, indications of long-term abuse)

Desired outcome: Family states an understanding of need for prompt medical care; family can state strategies learned from participation in parenting and stress management classes.

Diagnosis: Impaired home maintenance management related to inability of family members or caretakers to provide a safe home environment, as evidenced by multiple-injury pattern of presenting child; family denial of knowledge of presenting injuries

Desired outcome: Family states alternatives for child care and stress management; the child is provided a safe environment outside the family home until other resources can be initiated.

Diagnosis: *Potential for injury to the child related to maturational age of child and ineffective coping pattern of mother; impaired home maintenance pattern of family*

Desired outcome: The child experiences no further injury from caretaker(s).

Diagnosis: *Alteration in parenting related to inability of the caretaker(s) to provide a constructive environment which nurtures the growth and development of the child, as evidenced by long-term abuse of the child; developmental delays of the child*

Desired outcome: Family develops an awareness of the child's capabilities through parenting classes; parents verbalize acceptance of the child's right to be an individual.

Child Diagnoses

Diagnosis: *Impaired physical mobility related to limited physical movement from pain, as evidenced by multiple contusions, laceration, and swelling of left thigh; unable to sit, stand, or hold head up without assistance*

Desired outcome: Child maintains or resumes full mobility.

Diagnosis: *Powerlessness related to lack of personal control over certain events or situations, as evidenced by child's inability to protect or demand protection from abuse*

Desired outcome: Child states that it is alright to say someone is hurting him; child states what are good touches and what are bad touches.

Diagnosis: *Impairment of skin integrity related to contusions, laceration, and swelling of thigh with subsequent limited mobility*

Desired outcome: The child's skin heals without complications.

Diagnosis: *Disturbance in self-concept related to abusive parenting behavior in which child could experience or is at risk of experiencing a negative state in how he feels, thinks, or views himself, as evidenced by the feeling of abused children that "I must be bad or they wouldn't hurt me."*

Desired outcome: The child states that he is not the guilty party; the child states an understanding of the fact that parents were unable to cope; the child develops a positive concept of himself.

Child abuse and neglect occur in all classes and cultures where economic instability, isolation, unprepared parenthood, social stress, parent self-hate, a misplaced sexual drive, and/or inability to cope with the pressures of everyday life are factors. Regardless of the motivation, a child who is physically or mentally abused will be emotionally scarred for life, if the child survives.

Child abuse is a medical emergency, not just a social problem. Medical personnel have a unique opportunity to detect and report suspected abuse and neglect. Protection can then be provided for the child and help initiated for the parents. Again, it is not the responsibility of the ED personnel to obtain a definitive diagnosis of abuse or neglect. However, if there is any suspicion on the part of the provider, prompt care, documentation, and reporting are essential.

SUGGESTED READINGS

Ellerstein S: The cutaneous manifestations of child abuse and neglect. *Am J Dis Child* 1979;133:906–909.

Helfer RE, Kempe CH: Child abuse and neglect. The family and the community. Cambridge: Ballinger, 1976.

Johnson C, Coury D: Bruising and hemophilia. *Child Abuse Negl Int J* (in press).

Johnson C, Showers J: Injury variables in child abuse. *Child Abuse Negl* 1985;9:207–215.

Lenoski D, Hunter S: Specific patterns of inflicted burn injuries. *Trauma* 1977;17(11):842–846.

Morris J et al.: To report or not to report: physicians attitudes toward discipline and child abuse. *Am J Disease Child* 1985;139:194–197.

O'Hare AE, Eden OB: Bleeding disorders and non-accidental injury. *Arch Dis Child* 1984;59:860–864.

Rosenberg N et al.: Prediction of child abuse in an ambulatory setting. *Pediatrics* 1982; 70(6):879–882.

U.S. National Center on Child Abuse and Neglect: Child abuse and neglect: The problem and its management, an overview of the problem. Washington, D.C.: U.S. Government Printing Office. 1976: 38–39.

U.S. National Center on Child Abuse and Neglect: Child abuse and neglect: The problem and its management. The community team and approach to case management and prevention. Washington, D.C.: U.S. Government Printing Office. 1976:98–99.

Wilson T: Estimation of the age of cutaneous contusions in child abuse. *Pediatrics.* 1977;72(5):750–752.

8.2 ELDER ABUSE: INEFFECTIVE COPING

Carol A. Brown, MSW, LCSW

Mrs. B. presents to the ED with complaints of facial bruising and hip pain. She states she had fallen at home while washing dishes. Mrs. B. is well known to the staff; she is evaluated often for episodes of chest pain and shortness of breath with no known etiology. She has a primary physician who monitors her medications and is informed of each of her visits. During this visit, Mrs. B. is noted to have several areas of ecchymoses covering her abdomen and upper right chest area. Second-degree burns are seen on her thighs and lower abdomen. Her vital signs are within normal limits. She describes a moderate amount of pain.

Triage Assessment, Acuity Level IV: second-degree burns of abdomen and thighs.

Mrs. B. was taken immediately to the treatment area for management of her burns and evaluation of her other injuries. When Mrs. B. was determined to be stable and comfortable, the staff focused on her social history to determine more about the cause of her injuries.

Mrs. B. is a 79-year-old, white, divorced female who married at 16 years of age and conceived seven children. She moved to another state after her divorce, without the younger children (ages 10 and 12). Within 6 months, she returned to take the children with her, including the daughter who is now an adult and cares for her. Mrs. B. is retired; she suffered an MI and a CVA 2 years ago.

Mrs. B. led an active life until her CVA. Her family then noticed a deterioration in her strength and a personality change. Mrs. B. became depressed and would become emotional over simple problems. Although rehabilitation had enabled her to gain strength to walk, she was unable to drive. This was a source of great anguish for Mrs. B.

On past visits, Mrs. B. had confided to the nursing staff that she was unhappy at home. She depended on her daughter more and more for assistance with bathing, cleaning, and laundry. Mrs. B. said that she felt like a burden to her family. Her son leaves home for periods of time; her daughter works during the day, and Mrs. B. is unsupervised. Mrs. B. admitted her son drinks heavily and her daughter is upset over Mrs. B.'s grandson leaving home to join the military. Social work referrals had been offered, but Mrs. B. refused.

During this visit, the nursing staff suspected abuse. The physician and primary nurse questioned Mrs. B. regarding her injuries. She became anxious and tearful, requesting to be discharged. The primary nurse had established a relationship with Mrs. B. and explored the home situation further. Mrs. B. admitted that her daughter had thrown hot water at her because she could not rise from a chair. Also, Mrs. B. had slipped during a bathing incident, and her daughter had struck her.

The primary nurse and physician concluded that Mrs. B. was in an unsafe environment. A referral was made to the ED social worker and contact was made with the daughter. Initially, the daughter denied the incidents but later admitted that she was overwhelmed. The social worker contacted protective services and the primary nurse discussed community supports and the need for education regarding care. The medical team admitted Mrs. B. to the hospital to allow respite for the daughter and to evaluate the patient's injuries further. Follow-up support would be made by the inpatient staff.

QUESTIONS AND ANSWERS

1. What is elder abuse?

The number of elderly persons older than 75 years of age increases each year and has begun to constitute a significant percentage of the population. Innovative medical technology has increased the life span of those individuals over 65 years old. Yet this group presents with a new, complex set of problems (1,2). The elderly are often frail and vulnerable to a higher incidence of disease and multiple health problems (2).

There is no standard definition for elder abuse. Definitions vary widely and lack uniformity because it encompasses a wide variety of behaviors, conditions, and circumstances (3). Prevalence has also been difficult to quantify because of the reluctance of the elderly and the caregivers to accept the seriousness of the problem. Victims are not likely to admit that their caregiver is responsible for their injuries or neglected condition (2,4). This makes it equally difficult for health care providers to assess an elder abuse case. Also, health care providers share in their own sense of denial of the problem, lack of awareness of the problem, ageism, and insufficient knowledge of supportive resources (2,4).

Studies reveal there are an estimated 500,000 to 2.5 million victims (3). The wide range can be attributed to the problems of definition. More recent surveys suggest that there are 1.5 million cases (2). Victims cross all races, socioeconomic status, and ethnic origin (4).

The Elder Abuse Prevention, Identification and Treatment Act of 1985 defines abuse as

> . . . the willful infliction of injury, unreasonable confinement, intimidation or cruel punishment with resulting physical harm or pain or anguish; or the willful deprivation by a caretaker of goods or services which are necessary to avoid physical harm, mental anguish, or mental illness; the term 'exploitation' means the illegal or improper act or process of a caretaker using the resources of an elder for monetary or personal benefit, profit, or gain; the term 'neglect' means the failure to provide . . . the goods or services which are necessary to avoid physical harm, mental anguish or mental illness or the failure of a caregiver to provide such goods or services. The term 'physical harm' means bodily pain, injury, impairment or disease (5).

Three categories of elder abuse are defined for identification: physical harm, neglect, and mistreatment (3). Physical abuse is the deliberate physical contact that harms or intends to harm the individual. Neglect is the failure to provide necessary treatment and services for maintaining health and safety. Mistreatment is defined as the use of isolation, medications, or physical and chemical restraints with intent to harm. Mistreatment is most indicative of a psychological deficiency in the abuser (1,3,6).

National and state emphasis is placed on prevention and intervention with lawmakers amending the Older Americans Act to include definitions and funding. States now have mandatory reporting laws and reporting requirements. Legislation is still developing slowly. Many researchers feel elder abuse has emerged through the 1960's interest in child abuse and the 1970's interest in spouse abuse (7,8). Most of the reporting statutes include capabilities for immediate investigation and possible removal of the victim from the home in an emergency situation (4). Caseworkers from a protective services agency will conduct home assessments and will provide continuation of services and coordination for supportive measures. Inherent in this process is the patient's right to accept or refuse service. What is the victim's role in the decision-making process for his or her care and protection? Is the patient competent to make this decision? If yes, the victim has the right to refuse services. If there is a question of competency and ability to make rational decisions, measures will be taken to seek guardianship. These legal processes may protect and safeguard the person and property of the individual, but it is important to note that in some instances they can be tools of exploitation (6). Continued use of scientific studies to obtain empirical evidence of needs, prevalence, definition, and resources will validate and improve the care to the abused elderly.

Profiles of the victim and abuser are appearing in the literature that serve as valuable information for identifying and screening high-risk cases. A typically abused elder is over 75 years old, female, frail, and multiply dependent, who presents with several medical complaints. These medical problems impair the elder from caring for his or her own daily needs. Depression often occurs as the elder becomes more dependent. The individual requires assistance with activities of daily living, monitoring of medications, and management of finances (2,4,7).

The abuser is described as a family member, overwhelmed by the care demands and usually suffering from some type of stress. For example, nonresolution of a life crisis, substance abuse, unemployment, or poor family relationships (2,4,7). Percentages reveal that 40% are spouses of their victims; 50% are children or grandchildren (2,4).

Several theories have been postulated to explain the phenomenon of elder abuse. The impairment theory proposes that the elder is limited by a physical or mental disability that forces him or her to be dependent. The theory of psychopathology of the abuser contends that the abuser has personality traits or disorders that cause them to be abusive. Finally, the third theory is the stressed caregiver theory. Emphasis is placed on the burden of the caregiver to meet demands of the elder. Abuse will manifest itself as the internal pressures of frustration and resentment fuel and explode within the abuser. Not just one, but several of these theories can apply in one case (1).

Of note is the incidence of violence as a cyclical behavior pattern in the family. This pattern appears to be learned behavior that is accepted as a normal reaction to stress (1). The caretaker may have been abused as a child and may have observed other means of violence in the family (spouse abuse). In screening for abuse, it is important to realize that one family's mechanism for communicating may be a different exchange than what the health care provider expects or perceives to be normal. Further assessment and investigation is needed before a clear diagnosis can be made.

2. **What indicators lead to the assessment and identification of Mrs. B. as an abused elder?**

The detection of elder abuse is difficult. Victims most commonly present with complaints of medical problems (3,4). Psychological abuse appears more frequently than physical abuse; however, other studies reveal that psychological abuse with neglect will also often be accompanied by some type of physical abuse (3). Physical indicators are the most obvious and can range from signs of observable physical neglect to physical injury (2). Examples are unexplained injuries such as bruises, burns, and fractures; lack of supervision; constant hunger; poor hygiene; and unattended physical problems or medical needs (1). Neglect of a passive nature is the most common form of abuse (5,6). Neglect occurs when the caretaker fails to meet their obligation and the elder suffers from lack of food, attention, supervision, and abandonment.

Behavioral indicators provide information on the relationship between the caretaker and the elderly individual. An evasive or tearful response from an elderly person or no answer at all to questions regarding injury may be a clue to a risk situation (9). Excessive fear or paranoia in the presence of the caretaker may indicate an abusive situation (2,4). The caretaker's behavior is an alert to how the elderly person is treated. The nurse should carefully watch the interaction between the caretaker and elder. Although abusive language is normal in some families, it is important to follow-up on suspicions.

If the caretaker exhibits an obsession with control, reluctance for the elder to be evaluated in private, hostility toward the elder, improbable explanations for injuries, frustration at the burdens of caring for the individual, and has provided care for an extended length of time, abuse may be occurring. If the caretaker describes other problems that are causing stress such as illness, family dysfunction, unemployment, or alcohol or drug abuse, then the elder may be at risk (2,4,9).

To make a complete assessment, access to the home is necessary. Since this is not possible by nurses who work in acute care settings such as the ED, questions can be asked to determine if environmental indicators are present. For example, locks on the elder's bedroom door, kitchen, and bathroom are signs. Where is the patient's bedroom in relation to other family members? Is there access to the phone? Are there steps in the home that act as a barrier (2,4)? If there is need, does the elder have access to ambulation aids? Does the elder take a lot of medication, especially for sleep (4)?

Mrs. B. presented with several of these indicators. The combination of Mrs. B.'s bruising to the face, abdomen, and chest area plus the untreated burns were alert signs for the nurse. Mrs. B.'s frequent visits to the ED with complaints of unfounded chest pain and shortness of breath also were indicators. She lived at home with her children, and her care demands had exceeded the family's ability to provide care for her. The son had begun to leave the home, and supervision of care was placed upon the daughter. The son had begun to drink heavily; the daughter's son had left home and she was grieving the loss of that relationship. Mrs. B. had several injuries evident of trauma that had not received medical care. Assessment and recognition of these indicators assisted the nursing staff in diagnosing potential abuse which initiated further intervention.

3. **What are good effective exploratory questions that can be asked at the patient interview that may help illicit information that would clarify whether abuse has occurred?**

Particular questions to address that would be helpful in making a diagnosis of abuse are listed below:

Observations:

1. How severe is the patient's condition? Consider internal injuries.
2. Is the family cooperative with staff?
3. How do the patient and caregiver interact?
4. Is the home safe for the elder to return to?
5. How did the patient respond to talking to someone else?

Questions:

1. How did you receive your bruises?
2. When did this incident occur?
3. Why did you not seek medical care?
4. Can you ambulate well at home? Can you perform activities of daily living?
5. Were you alone when this happened? Who takes care of you?
6. Do you live alone or spend a lot of time alone?
7. Could your situation at home be improved?
8. Are there problems with your family? Illness? Drugs?
9. How do you think your caregiver feels about you?
10. Where do you go for routine medical care and follow-up?
11. Would your family be upset to know you are here and talking to me?

In the case of Mrs. B., the nurse did follow this guideline of questions. Information obtained allowed the staff to prepare a safe plan for Mrs. B. and her care.

4. **What are the nursing diagnoses appropriate to the phenomenon of elder abuse?**

Nursing diagnoses that are pertinent to the family cluster that suggest potential for abuse are those of relating and choosing. There are diagnoses pertinent to the family dynamics at large and those that relate to the individual victim of abuse.

Diagnosis: *Altered family processes related to the change in family roles of the patient's son and daughter because of the patient's poor health.*

Desired outcome: The patient's son and daughter will demonstrate more positive coping strategies when faced with stressful situations; the patient's son and daughter will acknowledge change in family roles and will participate in decisions regarding follow-up care.

Diagnosis: *Ineffective, compromised family coping related to insufficient, ineffective, and compromised support, comfort, assistance, and encouragement from the son and daughter to the mother to manage and master adaptive tasks related to her current health status*

Desired outcome: The patient's son and daughter will assist the patient to achieve maximum potential in performing self-care activities; the son and daughter will acknowledge needs of the patient and needs of the family as a unit; the family will participate in the treatment plan.

Diagnosis: *Self-esteem disturbance of the patient related to changes in health status, loss of independence, and dysfunctional behavior of the son and daughter.*

Desired outcome: The patient will verbalize more optimistic feelings of worth and seek to maximize her potential in her current health state.

Diagnosis: *Social isolation of the patient related to change in health status and dysfunctional behaviors of the son and daughter.*

Desired outcome: The patient and family will seek means to integrate the patient into social settings suited to current health state. Son and daughter will develop means to actively include patient in family affairs.

Diagnosis: *Impaired home maintenance management related to patient's decreased motor functioning and ineffective support mechanisms provided by the daughter and son.*

Desired outcome: The patient will be assisted by her son and daughter to achieve her potential in managing tasks at home independently, as possible; the patient's daughter and son will agree on ways to effectively cope with increased demands related to patient's home care.

Diagnosis: *Powerlessness of patient related to patient's pattern of helplessness from change in health status and feeling of dependence on her son and daughter for care.*

<u>Desired outcome:</u>   The patient will describe feeling in control. The patient will participate in decision making regarding her plan of care; the patient will share her feelings with her son and daughter.

5. **What intervention strategies should be developed in caring for Mrs. B.?**

Once abuse and/or neglect is identified, interventions will depend on the nature of the abuse or neglect, the setting, and the amount of information available (2). Nurses, physicians, social workers, and law enforcement personnel are the first line of defense for victims (6). Of all medical personnel, the nurse is most likely to be present when an elder needs help in sorting feelings. The nurse's activities can create an atmosphere where the patient feels free to reveal difficulties at home (10).

Complete information should be obtained regarding the patient's physical condition and documented specifically in the medical record (8). It is best to talk to the patient in private. Discuss with the patient the concerns and the willingness of staff to help improve the situation (8). It is important to recognize the needs of both the victim and caretaker; intervention must be directed at the well-being of the victim, but also to the coping ability of the abuser (8). The nurse should help the patient and family develop a plan that will improve the patient's care in the home or make alternative living arrangements. Focus should be on practical issues; what does the patient want? The nurse should provide the necessary psychosocial supports for the abuser with emphasis on skills training and self-managing training for the elderly (2,4,8).

A referral must be made to the welfare or social services agency responsible for follow-up. A protective services agency can initiate legal action against the abuser if necessary or provide interventions within the home environment (8). Interventions may include exploring alternative living arrangements, provision of in-home supports, supportive counseling, education and skills training for the abuser, and continued case management. Home health nurses are in a unique position to observe and monitor families in their home environment. They may be the first to identify a risk situation (9).

The nurse, in the case of Mrs. B., interviewed her separately from the daughter and consulted with the physician for further assessment. The nurse explored the home situation in a safe environment for the patient to verbalize her feelings. Mrs. B. began to present a clear profile of an abused elder. A referral was made to the ED social worker who referred the case to protective services and the inpatient worker for case management. The nurse responded to the needs of the daughter; continued interventions would be directed toward stabilizing the family and providing a safe environment for Mrs. B.

6. **What is the interface between nursing, social work, and physician intervention?**

Medical caretakers in acute-care settings are confronted with the increasing social problem of elder abuse. No one provider or profession should be responsible for the identification and management of these cases. A multidisciplinary team should be used whenever possible. The team can include physicians, nurses, social workers, attorneys, and psychiatrists. Specified goals are for coordination, education, diagnosis, treatment, consultation, and prevention (1,2,3). Teams will vary because of local resources and the structure of the institution. Since the elderly are more difficult to care for, physicians will have to spend more time and patience to provide treatment. Social workers are challenged to uphold the rights of the elderly yet adhere to the requirements of the legal system. Many of the issues involved with elder abuse are of a social nature. Nurses are in a position to be present when the patient is most vulnerable and willing to sort out their feelings. Establishing a reputation as a helping professional allows the nurse the advantage of performing ongoing assessments. Nurses are usually the first responder to care, whether it is through triage or acute care.

The case of Mrs. B. would be appropriate for staff case conference. Increasing awareness among nursing staff of elder abuse would provide knowledge and understanding when other cases present.

REFERENCES

1. Fulmer T: Elder abuse. In: Abuse and victimization across the life span. Straus MB, ed. Baltimore: University Press, 1988: 188.

2. Council on Scientific Affairs: Elder abuse and neglect. *JAMA* 1987; 257:966.

3. Matlaw J. Mayer J: Elder abuse: ethical and practical dilemmas for social work. *Health Soc Work* May, 1986:85.

4. Taler G: Elder abuse. *Fam Phys* 1985; 32:107.

5. Trilling J, Greenblatt DO, Shephard C: Elder abuse and utilization of support services for elderly patients. *J Fam Pract* 1987;24:581.

6. Douglass R: Domestic mistreatment of the elderly—towards prevention. Washington, DC: Criminal Justices Services/AARP, 1987:2.

7. Powills S: Elder abuse: what role do hospitals play? *Hospitals* 1988;62:84.

8. Bachur J, Lawrence F, Watson M: Elder abuse manual. Department of Social Work. Baltimore, Johns Hopkins Hospital. 1985:2.

9. Thobaben M: Abuse: the shameful secret of elder care. *RN* 1988;51:85.

10. Walke M: When a patient needs to unburden his feelings. *Am J Nurs* 1977; 6:1164.

CHAPTER 9
Emotional Health System

Overview

Behavioral outcomes and expressions of feelings based on an individual's perception of self (mind, body) as it interfaces with change in health status are evaluated in the emotional health system. The nursing assessment includes the capacity of the individual to draw on adaptive behaviors needed to maintain or regain homeostasis in response to life stressors.

Suicide attempts and aggressive behavior management are two highly intensive patient situations that are equally as stressful to the nurse and ED care providers as any emergent trauma presentation. The emotional drain on staff in these situations can be significant. The following two case studies provide strategies for nursing care that help to minimize poor outcomes for the patient while lending emotional support (control) to the staff.

CUE WORDS

BEHAVIOR	FEELINGS
adjustment	anxiety
coping	fear
diversional activities	grieving
posttrauma response	hopelessness
self-control	powerlessness
thought process	self-concept
violence	sexual self-concept
	gender identity
	spiritual distress

RELATED NURSING DIAGNOSES

body image disturbance
self-esteem disturbance
chronic low self-esteem
situational low self-esteem
personal identity disturbance
hopelessness
powerlessness
dysfunctional grieving
anticipatory grieving
potential for violence: self-directed or directed at others
post trauma response
rape—trauma syndrome
rape—trauma syndrome: compound reaction
rape—trauma syndrome: silent reaction
anxiety
fear

spiritual distress (distress of human spirit)
diversional activity deficit
ineffective denial
ineffective individual coping
impaired adjustment

Department of Emergency Medicine Triage Protocols

Emotional Health System

Level I	Level II	Level III	Level IV
Patient expresses sadness, dejection, unworthiness; feelings may be appropriate to reality; mild and/or transitory depression; no suicidal or homicidal ideation	Patient depressed with change in ADL, eating, or sleeping habits; somatic complaints; no suicidal or homicidal ideation; patient waiting with a responsible significant other	Same as I or II but has suicidal or homicidal ideation without a plan; patient will be waiting with a responsible significant other and can contract to safely wait in waiting room	Expresses suicidal or homicidal ideation with plan; thoughts may contain gross misrepresentation of reality; body and motor activity may be slowed and decreased or rapid and agitated
			Suicidal or homicidal gesture
Experiencing mild anxiety; not dysfunctional	Displays anxious behavior	Perceptual field is greatly reduced; attention may focus on a specific detail; can follow instructions with much direction	Loss of control; unable to do things even with direction; perceptions may be distorted; unable to communicate or function effectively
Mild, transient anger		Frustrated but able to control behavior; some contact with reality; will be waiting with a responsible significant other	Unable to control anger; perception of reality temporarily impaired by emotions; real or potential for injury to self or others
			All patients at risk for elopement
			All emergency petition patients

203

9.1 SUICIDE: ASSESSING RISK
Debra Lanouette, RN, MSN, CS

Ruth is a 25-year-old white female who was brought to the ED by her boyfriend after she cut her left wrist several times with a razor blade. She is disheveled in appearance, tearful, and obviously quite distressed. She admits to having cut her wrist in a suicide attempt after her boyfriend (of 6 months) came home intoxicated, began to argue with her, and told her he wanted to terminate the relationship. She went into the bathroom and cut herself several times before being discovered by her boyfriend.

She denies any premeditation of the suicide act or recent change in mood or behavior, although she has been worried about her boyfriend's heavy alcohol use. Ruth was born and raised in a large metropolitan area, graduated from high school in 1982, and currently works as a hairdresser. Her family history includes alcoholism in her father and an attempted suicide by a sister while "depressed." Three years ago, during a dispute with a boyfriend, Ruth took an overdose of 15 to 20 Tylenol tablets, was seen in the ED, and released. She has had no psychiatric hospitalizations or outpatient treatment. She admits to occasional use of marijuana and alcohol, usually on the weekends and often to the point of intoxication, but denies a history of blackouts or withdrawal. Her boyfriend was recently released from jail for burglary and has a history of alcoholism and spouse abuse.

Ruth is difficult to engage in conversation and avoids eye contact. She is tearful and describes feeling "very depressed." Her affect is sad and irritable. Her speech is normal in volume, rate, and rhythm and is logical and goal-directed; there is no evidence of a formal thought disorder. Cognitively she is alert and oriented x3, with a clear sensorium and no evidence of alcohol or drug use. She denies hallucinations, delusions, obsessions, compulsions, and phobias. She states cutting her wrist was "stupid"; she had not intended to die, rather she was in "a panic" at the thought of her boyfriend leaving her and "just wanted him to stop drinking." She denies current suicidal ideation and intent.

Triage Assessment, Acuity Level III: Suicidal behavior; no current ideation or immediate intent; patient will be waiting with a responsible family member and can contract to notify staff immediately should she experience a recurrence of suicidal thoughts or wish to leave the department before being seen by a physician.

QUESTIONS AND ANSWERS

1. **What are the current demographics of suicide? How does the nurse distinguish between the high-risk and low-risk suicidal patient?**

   ED nurses are frequently called upon to provide care to patients presenting with suicidal behaviors. Suicidal behaviors include the expression of suicidal ideation, suicide attempts, and completed suicides (1). Approximately 29,000 persons commit suicide each year in the United States, making it the eighth leading cause of death (2). It is estimated, however, that the rate of suicide attempts is at least 10 times the rate of completed suicides (3). It is well documented that while females attempt suicide 3:1 over males, males succeed 3 times as often as females (4). This success rate is related to more serious intent and more lethal means (firearms, hanging, etc.) used by males. White males 60 years and older represent the highest percentage of completed suicides, particularly when other risk factors are present such as failing health, loss of a spouse or significant other, isolation or weak social supports, and alcoholism (5).

Although the presence of depressive illness and/or alcoholism correlate highly with suicide, the most sensitive predictor of a serious attempt is the presence of hopelessness (6,7). The hopeless and helpless patient views his or her present anguish and despair as unending and is unable to see a way out of what is experienced as an unbearable existence. Patients at high risk for a lethal attempt generally have contemplated and planned their suicides over a period of time, may have gotten their affairs in order or prepared a suicide note, and execute their attempts under circumstances designed to minimize the chance of discovery or rescue.

In contrast to patients at risk for completed suicides are "suicide-attempters," who, like Ruth, tend to be female (2:1 over males), 20 to 30 years of age, with histories of unstable interpersonal relationships and employment patterns (2,8). The methods most frequently utilized in suicide attempts by these patients are pill overdose (70 to 90%) and wrist cutting (11%) (8). The suicide attempt is often precipitated by the perceived loss of a significant other and occurs impulsively, with low intent and low fatality risk. These attempts may be termed "parasuicides" or "object-related" attempts, as the intent is usually not so much to end one's life as to prevent abandonment or elicit a caring response from the significant other. In some individuals this can become a chronic behavioral response when similarly stressed. It must be emphasized, however, that *all* suicidal behaviors should be taken seriously, as it is entirely possible that an impulsive, low-intent attempt could result in a fatal outcome if the patient ingests a highly toxic agent (e.g., tricyclic antidepressants) or attempts hanging, shooting, or drowning.

In assessing suicide risk, the nurse must consider the broad clinical picture, the demographic profile, and the circumstances of the attempt. In particular, it must be elicited whether the patient intended to die, what the patient expected to happen, and whether the patient regrets having survived the attempt and will continue to have suicidal ideation or intent. A useful tool for analyzing the circumstances of a suicide attempt is Weisman's "Risk-Rescue Rating Scale" (9) which considers the agent used, its effect on the patient (level of consciousness, reversibility), and the chances of the patient being discovered and rescued. The evaluation of suicide risk is optimally made in collaboration with a psychiatrist or other well-trained psychiatric professional.

2. **Are there any personality traits or characteristics that predispose a patient to object-related suicide attempts (parasuicide)?**

Although there is no clearly defined "suicidal personality," there are historical and characterological features that may contribute to a pattern of suicide attempts. These patients have often been reared in unstable or chaotic families where parental figures were insensitive or unresponsive to the patient's emotional needs and thus made the development of healthy attachment behaviors impossible. Alcoholism in one or both parents is a common finding (10). In addition, these patients may have suffered neglect, physical abuse, or sexual abuse. As adults these individuals tend to be needy and dependent in their relationships and are extremely sensitive to the retreat or potential abandonment by their partners. They view themselves as bad, unlovable, and unloved, often choosing partners who are themselves unstable, abusive, and unable to make healthy and mature emotional attachments. The patient may exhibit characterological traits suggestive of a personality disorder or may meet the diagnostic criteria necessary to formally make the diagnosis. Patients with borderline personality disorder are frequently seen in EDs with suicidal ideation or following a self-destructive act. Gunderson (11) has identified the essential features of this disorder, which include intense, unstable interpersonal relationships; unstable sense of self; negative affects; impulsivity; and low achievement. He points out that self-destructive behavior is extremely prevalent in the disorder, generally manifested in self-mutilation or "manipulative" suicide attempts, sexual promiscuity, reckless behavior, and alcohol or drug abuse. Suicide attempts are usually in response to anticipated loss which arouses intensely dysphoric affects including panic, rage, and helplessness. These patients may be extremely fearful of being alone, having tenuous sense of self, and perceive rejection and abandonment by a partner as not only loss of the relationship, but a loss of the self.

3. **What nursing diagnoses are applicable in this situation?**

Nursing diagnoses for the patient who has attempted suicide should consider the patient's physical and psychological needs.

Diagnosis: Impaired skin integrity related to self-inflicted lacerations of the wrist

Desired patient outcome: The patient will have cessation of bleeding from the wound; the patient will verbalize an understanding of wound care; the patient will not experience a wound infection.

Diagnosis: ***Self-directed violence related to feelings of powerlessness and fear of abandonment***

Desired patient outcome: The patient will express no suicidal ideation or intent; the patient identifies and agrees to a well-defined plan for managing suicidal ideation in the future.

Diagnosis: ***Ineffective individual coping related to feelings of help-lessness and inadequacy***

Desired patient outcome: The patient identifies alternative, more adaptive coping strategies; the patient identifies mental health resources and voices a willingness to participate in treatment.

4. What medical interventions would likely take place, and what nursing interventions should the nurse initiate in this situation?

All laceration wounds should be cleaned with a mild antiseptic soap or hydrogen peroxide and then irrigated with normal saline. Ruth's lacerations were sutured by the surgeon with 4.0 dermalon x4. An antibiotic ointment may be applied, followed by the application of a sterile dressing. The nurse should administer tetanus-diphtheria toxoid if the patient has not received one within the past 5 years. Oral antibiotics are not generally prescribed, although a local antibiotic ointment may be. The nurse should review wound and dressing care and the date to return for suture removal with the patient.

Depending on the setting and care delivery system, the nurse may play an integral role in collaborating with a psychiatrist or mental health professional in evaluating suicide risk. All psychiatric patients should be questioned directly about suicidal ideation or intent, including how seriously suicide has been contemplated, whether a plan has been formulated, and whether the patient has the means to execute the plan. The patient and family should be questioned about changes in behavior that indicate an impending suicide attempt, i.e., withdrawal from usual activities and significant others, putting affairs in order or making out a will, or giving away valued possessions. A past history of suicide attempts or family history of psychiatric illness or suicide should be elicited. It is also critical that the nurse assess the patient for the risk of an *immediate* self-destructive act or suicide attempt in the ED. The question should be asked, "Do I need to be concerned that you will try to harm yourself here in the ED?" Patients exhibiting (or with histories of) impulsivity, self-destructiveness, low frustration tolerance, and anger toward care providers should be considered at risk. This is particularly true if the patient is intoxicated (alcohol is a disinhibitor). In the patient who has made a suicide attempt the intent and seriousness of the attempt should be elicited. The patient should be asked if there is any regret that the attempt was unsuccessful and whether there is continued suicidal ideation or intent.

Patients who express suicidal ideation or intent, and those who have attempted suicide, especially if assessed as representing an immediate risk for a self-destructive act in the ED, should be searched and any potentially dangerous items removed from that person. Although every effort should be made to not unduly violate a patient's right to privacy and autonomy, the nurse has an overriding duty to protect from harm those patients believed to be at risk for injury to self or others (12). The nurse should approach the patient in a calm, respectful, and nonthreatening manner, perhaps saying, "I need to check your pockets and purse to make sure you are safe." The patient may then be less resistant to being searched. The patient must also be placed on suicide precautions, which generally means placing the patient in a highly visible and well-lighted location where he or she may be observed on a one-to-one basis. Patients should be accompanied to the bathroom. Family members cannot be permitted to assume responsibility for this observation.

The nurse must be aware of his or her own emotional responses to suicide attempters, especially anger, indifference, hate, or helplessness. It is essential that the nurse maintain an objective and professional response and control emotional reactivity, as these patients are often acutely sensitive to perceived disinterest or rejection on the part of the care provider. A therapeutic alliance should be established between the patient and a small, stable number of care providers, so as to minimize the patient's attempts to manipulate or "split" staff. When managing patients with borderline personality disorder, Cousins (13) also emphasizes giving clear directions and expectations, providing structure, and focusing on the task at hand. A consistent approach by all providers is essential.

The nurse may provide brief crisis-oriented intervention, focusing on the precipitating event or stressors, the feelings aroused or emotional response, and the patient's usual coping strategies. The maladaptive strategy of suicide attempting must be identified as such and alternatives explored. It should be pointed out that this behavior may in fact anger or repulse the significant other, diminishing even further the chance that they will remain in the relationship. The nurse should verbalize hope that the patient can develop more healthy and adaptive means of getting emotional needs met. Efforts should be made to identify and mobilize social support systems.

The psychiatrist or mental health professional will conduct a formal psychiatric interview, including a social, psychiatric, and medical history, and mental status exam. Based on this evaluation they will determine whether or not a psychiatric illness is present and a DSMIII-R (Diagnostic and Statistical Manual III-Revised) diagnosis will be made. They will decide if the patient can receive psychiatric care on an outpatient basis or if psychiatric hospitalization is necessary. For patients believed to be at risk for a suicide attempt and who refuse voluntary psychiatric hospitalization, the psychiatrist or mental health professional will determine whether the patient meets the criteria for involuntary hospitalization (certification) and will initiate the process.

In this case, the psychiatrist made the following DSMIII-R diagnoses: Adjustment disorder with disturbance in mood and conduct and R/O (rule out) borderline personality disorder. The psychiatrist and nurse collaborated in providing brief crisis-oriented intervention, following which the patient expressed an improved mood and no further suicidal ideation. The patient expressed a willingness to participate in outpatient treatment and a referral was made to her local Community Mental Health Center. She was able to identify several alternative strategies for coping with anger and dysphoria and agreed to call or return to the ED should she experience serious suicidal ideation or intent.

REFERENCES

1. Beck AT, Davis JH, Frederick CJ et al.: Classification and nomenclature in suicide prevention in the Seventies, In: Suicide Prevention in the Seventies ed. by H. Resnick and B. Hawthorne (Washington, DC: US Government Printing Office), p. 7–12.

2. Hirschfeld R, Davidson L: Risk factors for suicide. In: Frances AJ, Hales RE, eds. Review of Psychiatry, vol. 7. Washington, D.C.: American Psychiatric Press, 1988.

3. Davidson LE: Study of suicide attempts during a cluster of suicides. Paper presented at the Epidemic Intelligence Service Conference, Atlanta, 1986.

4. Pellitier LR, Cousins A: Clinical assessment of the suicidal patient in the emergency department. *J Emerg Nurs* 1984; 10:40–43.

5. Osgood N: Suicide in the elderly, Rockville, MD: Aspen Systems Corporation, 1985.

6. Beck AT et al.: Hopelessness and eventual suicide: A ten year prospective study of patients hospitalized with sui-

cidal ideation. *Am J Psychiatry* 1985; 142:539–563.

7. Fawcett J et al.: Clinical predictors of suicide in patients with major affective disorders: A controlled prospective study. *Am J Psychiatry* 1987;144: 35–40.

8. Jacobs D: Evaluation and care of suicidal behavior in emergency settings. *Int J Psychiatry Med* 1983;12:295–308.

9. Weisman AD, Worden JW: Risk-rescue rating in suicide assessment. *Arch Gen Psychiatry* 1979;30:555–560.

10. Stephens BJ: Cheap thrills and humble pie: The adolescence of female suicide attempters. *Suicide Life Threat Behav* 1987;17:107–119.

11. Gunderson J: Borderline personality disorder. Washington, D.C.: American Psychiatric Press, 1984.

12. Driscoll K: Search and seizure in the emergency department. *J Emerg Nurs* 1986;12:76–80.

13. Cousins A: Management of the emergency department patient with a borderline personality disorder. *J Emerg Med* 1984;10:94–96.

9.2 AGGRESSIVE BEHAVIOR MANAGEMENT
Debra Lanouette, RN, MSN, CS

Mrs. T. is a 31-year-old white female who is escorted by the police to the ED with an emergency petition. According to her sister, Ms. K., the patient has not slept in 3 days, is talking constantly, and is argumentative and threatening. Mrs. T. has been leaving the house during the night and walking around the neighborhood for 2 to 4 hr at a time. She has not eaten in 2 days claiming "I don't need food; food is for mortals."

Mrs. T. is large and disheveled, appears to be her stated age, and looks well nourished. She is following directions and, in fact, is quite gregarious, smiling and extending her hand to all persons nearby, introducing herself as "Medea, a prophet of God." Mrs. T. describes her mood as "great, terrific." Her affect is labile, and at times markedly irritable. Her speech is loud, rapid, and pressured, with loosening of associations. She will give her proper name with encouragement and is oriented to place and time. She is alert, appears cognitively intact, and there are no fluctuations in her level of consciousness. She openly and vividly reports hearing "the voice of God" who tells her she is a messenger who has the power "to save our culture from certain doom." She is seductive and hypersexual with the male security personnel. Her vital signs are temperature 98.8°F, pulse 90, respirations 20, and BP 130/76. Her past psychiatric records establish a prior diagnosis of bipolar disorder, manic phase.

Triage Assessment, Acuity Level IV: Emergency Petition.

QUESTIONS AND ANSWERS

1. **What patients are most at risk for aggressive behavior in the ED?**

All too frequently nurses in the ED are called upon to manage patients who are verbally abusive, threatening, or physically aggressive. These behaviors can arouse strong feelings in care providers including fear, vulnerability, anger, and inadequacy. Prompt recognition of escalating patient behavior and early, appropriate intervention can, however, minimize the risk of injury to the patient, staff, and others.

Aggressive behavior occurs when stimuli, either internal or external, overwhelm the individual, producing intense fear and a sense of threat and powerlessness. There is frequently a weakening of the patient's internal controls. Risk factors for aggressive behavior include a history of violence, particularly violence that has occurred immediately prior to arrival in the ED, and violent family or social systems. Drug and alcohol abuse can significantly contribute to agitated, threatening behavior. Alcohol particularly acts as a disinhibitor.

Psychiatric (functional) disorders associated with aggression include schizophrenia (paranoid type), bipolar disorder (mania), and personality disorder (borderline, antisocial type). Aggressive behavior in the acutely psychotic patient is often in response to frightening hallucinations, delusions, and impaired reality-testing. These produce terrifying feelings of threat and vulnerability. The patient's aggressive response tends to be diffuse and nonfocused and is intended to protect the individual from what is perceived as immediate danger. In contrast, patients with a personality disorder manifest life-long characterological traits that predispose them to volatile behavior. These include poor frustration tolerance, impulsivity, self-destructiveness, and anger towards care providers. Threatening or aggressive behavior in these individuals is most likely to occur if the care provider is perceived as aloof, rejecting, or disinterested, or when the "agenda" of the patient is not met, i.e., the physician refuses to give a prescription drug of abuse. The volatile outbursts of personality disorder patients tend to be more focused and at times willful and malicious.

Patients with medical illnesses, including conditions that may be life-threatening, may present with "psychiatric symptoms," including agitated or violent behavior. The most common conditions in the emergency setting include acute alcohol and/or drug intoxication or withdrawal, head trauma, seizure disorders, cerebral tumors, and organic brain syndromes including delirium, and dementia (1). An organic etiology should be suspected in any patient who is age 40 or older with no history of psychiatric illness, who has experienced a rapid change in mental state and presents with disorientation, clouded sensorium, alteration in level of consciousness, and abnormal vital signs.

2. **Are patients with bipolar disorder, manic phase, more at risk for aggressive behavior than other patients with major mental illness?**

Not necessarily. However, an acutely manic patient is more likely to "fool" care providers, who are seduced by his or her gregarious and entertaining demeanor and may relax their clinical guard against the threat of physical harm.

Bipolar disorder is characterized by cyclical disturbances in mood and behavior. Usually there are depressive and manic cycles, although in 10 to 20% of all cases there are only manic episodes (2). Mean age of onset is 30 years, although it can occur anytime between childhood and age 50. There is strong evidence for a genetic or biologic basis for bipolar disorder, although psychosocial factors may also play a role in its etiology. Bipolar disorder is a life-long problem, requiring ongoing psychiatric care and treatment. Lithium is the drug of choice for this disorder, although neuroleptics may be needed during manic episodes. Medication noncompliance is a significant factor in relapse and ED visits.

The acutely manic patient experiences an elevated mood, enormous energy, heightened self-esteem and sense of power, and may have auditory or visual hallucinations and grandiose delusions. The patient is generally restless, loud, and hyperverbal with rapid, pressured speech, and disorganization of thought.

There is often pronounced mood lability with an underlying irritability that can emerge quickly. The patient can become threatening, verbally abusive, or violent, particularly when limits are set or when psychiatric hospitalization is discussed. A degree of clinical reserve is *always* necessary when caring for acutely manic patients.

3. **What nursing diagnoses are applicable in this situation?**

    Diagnosis: Potential for violence, directed at self and others, related to psychomotor hyperactivity, mood lability, overwhelming affects, and misinterpretation of reality

    Desired patient outcome: The patient will maintain or regain internal controls and not injure self or others; the patient will demonstrate a decrease in psychomotor hyperactivity; the patient will verbalize more adaptive strategies for managing overwhelming feelings of rage, frustration, fear, and powerlessness; the patient will distinguish between hallucinations and external events and demonstrate improved reality testing.

    Diagnosis: Noncompliance with medication regime related to knowledge deficit

    Desired patient outcome: The patient, family, and/or significant others will verbalize an understanding of bipolar disorder and the need for long-term psychiatric treatment and medication.

4. **What nursing interventions are most effective in managing aggressive patients?**

    Early recognition, intervention, and prevention are the keys to managing aggressive patients. Although these can be difficult to achieve in a busy emergency setting where patients sometimes arrive wildly out of control, there are ways to manage an escalating or violent patient that minimize the risk of assault or injury to both the patient and the staff. The goals for managing aggressive patients include assisting the patient to maintain or regain internal controls and preventing injury to the patient, staff, and others.

    Smith (3) describes an assault cycle which, if recognized, can be interrupted by appropriate and timely intervention. This cycle begins with a trigger (internal or external). If unchecked, this trigger progresses to escalation. This escalation phase is characterized by increasing tension and volatility; a weakening of impulse control; and progression, if uninterrupted, toward aggression or assault. This phase may last minutes to several hours. The shortest but most intense period is the assault (crisis) phase, where the patient loses control and becomes acutely violent. Following an assault, the patient will usually de-escalate and eventually stabilize.

Interventions for the manic patient are outlined in accordance with Smith's model of the assault cycle (3). Appropriate clinical responses should be based on *where the patient is* in the assault cycle. At all times, however, the nurse should manage patients in a humane and concerned manner, using the least restrictive intervention that is consistent with patient and staff safety.

Activation

The nurse must be acutely sensitive to changes in patient behavior or signs of escalation. These cues include increased muscle tension, restlessness or pacing, clenched teeth or fists, an angry facial expression, and/or loud strident speech (4). Nursing interventions are as follows:

- *Acknowledge* the increased tension state; ask the patient to *talk* about what is occurring; giving the patient an opportunity to verbalize thoughts and feelings may decrease the need to act them out behaviorally
- Build a therapeutic alliance and elicit the cooperation of the patient; extend your hand and introduce yourself; let the patient know you are concerned and want to help; ask directly how you might help or what she can do for herself to feel more comfortable and maintain control.
- *Identify* and eradicate the triggering stimuli, if possible; ask the patient what is causing her to feel tense or restless; simple interventions, like asking an antagonistic family member to wait in the waiting room, may be all that is needed.
- Encourage involvement from family or friends; the presence of a supportive friend or family member may be enormously reassuring and calming.
- Offer food or liquids; this simple nurturant gesture conveys warmth and concern.
- Aid in reality testing; help the patient to distinguish between hallucinations or delusions and external reality.

Escalation

A patient who is becoming increasingly more agitated and threatening and is in tenuous control must be managed using a firm and highly directive approach. Nursing interventions during this phase are intended to halt the progression toward loss of control and assault.

- Acknowledge the increasing tension and threat to others; express the expectation that the patient remain in control and not hurt anyone; let her know you are there to assist with controls.

- Evaluate your risk by assessing your location; move out of an office or isolated area.
- Summon security personnel; sometimes a show of force will encourage a patient to remain in control; on the other hand it may sometimes provoke patients who feel threatened and need to "rise to the occasion" with physical aggressiveness; in any event it is best to have security respond and be available should violence erupt.
- Control your own emotional reactivity; there is nothing that will make a patient feel more anxious than a staff person who is apprehensive, emotionally reactive, or provocative.
- Provide clear directions, choices, and consequences; do not beg, plead, or bargain with the patient.
- Position yourself either greater than an arm's length away from the patient *or* very close in and to the side; avoid too intense eye contact.
- Use open-door seclusion if the patient is very stimulated, threatening, or in tenuous control; give a clear command and escort the patient in, if needed; clearly state the expectation that she remain in seclusion.
- Search any patient that may be dangerous to self or others and remove potentially harmful items (matches, belts, sharps); although every effort should be made to not unduly violate a patient's right to privacy and autonomy, a nurse has an overriding duty to protect a patient from harm (5).
- Offer oral psychotropic medications; high-potency neuroleptics (Haldol, Prolixin) in oral concentrate form are recommended for their ease of administration, rapid onset of action, and sedating effects; following administration observe the patient carefully for extrapyramidal side effects; acute dystonia is most prevalent in young males (6) and can lead to laryngospasm and respiratory distress. Dystonia can be treated successfully with intramuscular Benadryl or Cogentin (antiparkinsonian).

Assault

The patient at this point has lost control and is combative and violent. This patient requires rapid intervention with an organized team approach. Physical restraint may be necessary.

- Do not approach the patient until a team (at least two persons, optimally four to five) is assembled and ready to respond; one person should be the designated leader, giving direction to the other team members.
- Approach the patient diagonally; each team member should be assigned a limb to restrain; the team should use safe and humane restraint techniques, escorting the patient to seclusion and placing her

on a mat or restraining her to a stretcher (four-point restraints); locked-door seclusion may be necessary at this time.

• Continue talking to the patient, letting her know you are assuming control at this time to prevent injury to the patient and others; let her know what is happening, what the plan is, and that she is safe.

• Patients on emergency petition for psychiatric evaluation may be brought to the ED in handcuffs and/or foot shackles; assess the patient's control carefully and obtain vital signs before removing cuffs; elicit information from the officer about resistance or aggression during transport; remove cuffs in a seclusion room or after placing the patient on a stretcher; examine wrists and ankles carefully for fractures or soft tissue injury.

• Use universal precautions when coming into contact with blood or body fluids.

• If needed, administer high-potency neuroleptic medication intramuscularly for rapid tranquilization. Droperidol is a potent butyrophenone neuroleptic that is useful in the psychiatric emergency setting because of its rapid onset of action (< 5 min) (7) and relatively low incidence of extrapyramidal side effects (8). Droperidol can produce marked hypotension and is therefore contraindicated in patients with dehydration or a low baseline blood pressure. A benzodiazepine may be a safer alternative for the hypotensive patient and those who are extremely sensitive to the extrapyramidal side effects of neuroleptics.

Recovery and Stabilization

Recovery is the time period when the patient is de-escalating and regaining internal controls. Stabilization is achieved when the patient is in control, is calm and cooperative, and is amenable to treatment. The nurse should continue to assess the patient frequently, giving positive feedback for appropriate behavior, and gradually wean her from seclusion or restraints. Every effort should be made to stabilize a patient prior to transport to an outside facility.

5. **What disposition would be appropriate for this patient?**

Mrs. T. is having an acute exacerbation of her bipolar disorder, manic phase. She is safely managed in the ED using oral neuroleptics (Haldol) and open-door seclusion. Her lithium level of 0.2 mEq/liter (therapeutic range is 0.8 to 1.5 mEq/liter) suggests medication noncompliance. Psychiatric hospitalization is indicated to provide a safe, structured environment and restabilization of the patient with medications.

Mrs. T. agreed to come into the hospital voluntarily. If she had not, the psychiatrist would need to determine if the patient meets the criteria for involuntary hospitalization. The nurse and psychiatrist discussed with both the patient and her sister the nature of her disorder, and emphasized the need for long-term psychiatric outpatient care and compliance with medication.

REFERENCES

1. Slaby AW: Quality assurance and diagnostic psychiatry. In: Dubin WR, Hanke N, Nickens HW, eds. Psychiatric emergencies. New York: Churchill Livingstone, 1984.
2. Kaplan HI, Sadock BJ, eds.: Mood disorders, synopsis of psychiatry. Baltimore: Williams & Wilkins, 1988.
3. Smith P: Management of assaultive behavior (training manual). Sacramento, California: California Department of Developmental Services, 1977.
4. Dubin WR: Evaluating and managing the violent patient. *Ann Emerg Med* 1981;10(9):481–484.

5. Driscoll K: Search and seizure in the emergency department. *J Emerg Nurs* 1986;12:76–80.
6. Zavodnick S: Psychopharmacology. In: Dubin WR, Hanke N, Nickens HW, eds. Psychiatric emergencies. New York: Churchill Livingstone, 1984.
7. Hooper J, Minter G: Droperidol in the management of psychiatric emergencies. *J Clin Psychopharmacol* 1983;3: 262–263.
8. Resnick M, Burton B: Droperidol vs. haloperidol in the initial management of acutely agitated patients. *J Clin Psychiatry* 1984;45:298–299.

CHAPTER 10

Health Management System

Overview

The health management system encompasses the individual's motivation to manage personal health-related activities. The health management system includes a person's perception of his or her own health status and a person's motivation to strive for an optimal level of wellness as demonstrated by follow through with the therapeutic treatment plan. The patient's choices related to compliance are stressed in this parameter for the ED patient. As with patients who have inadequate support systems, these patient's social support and health maintenance needs are less acute than their physical needs in most instances. Nonetheless, the patient should not be discharged without some determination of ability or willingness to comply with the treatment plan, including an assessment of financial, intellectual, emotional, and social resources.

Two case studies selected for demonstration of patient care needs and nursing interventions within this health system address the issues of compliance and motivation.

CUE WORDS

COMPLIANCE	MOTIVATION
health maintenance	congruence with life-
health practices	style
life-style	health perception
self-care	incentive
smoking	needs assessment
substance use or	personal goals
abuse	

RELATED NURSING DIAGNOSES

impaired home maintenance management
altered health maintenance
noncompliance (specify)
health-seeking behaviors (specify)

Department of Emergency Medicine Triage Protocols

Health Management System

Level I	Level II	Level III	Level IV
Noncompliance with Rx regimen (meds, appts., diet), revealed on routine interview; nonsymptomatic	Noncompliance with Rx regimen is precipitating factor in this episode, e.g., wound infection, hypertension	Continued lack of compliance (deliberate or unintentional) would pose life-threatening situation, e.g., DKA, CHF, recurrent GI bleeds	
Does not use safety devices in hazardous environment—current visit is a product of this behavior	Repeatedly treated as a result of poor safety practices—current pattern is potentially self-destructive		
Identifies deficiencies in ADL; able to follow instructions and cooperate with intervention plan	Identifies problem with self-care but is unable or unwilling to cooperate in planned intervention	Presents with significant illness or injury secondary to self-care deficit, e.g., hypothermic, untreated ulcers	
	Presents unclean and unkempt, with infestation; inadequate clothing		
	Homeless, indigent, unable to access social service or health care system—refer to social worker		

Preexisting condition requires more in-depth care than patient or support system is able to mobilize

Presents because not accepted at other health program, i.e., substance abuse; unable to get shelter; detox.

10.1 HIGH BLOOD PRESSURE:
EDUCATION AND COMPLIANCE
Debra Kosko, MN, CRNP

Mr. Scott is a 51-year-old black male who arrived ambulatory into the ED triage area. He states that 20 min ago he picked up a drinking glass and it broke, lacerating his finger. A 1-cm superficial laceration of the patient's right fifth digit is noted by the triage nurse. The laceration area is cleansed and dressed, while the patient waits to be sutured. Mr. Scott's vital signs at triage are BP 174/114, pulse 76 and regular, respirations 20 and easy. Mr. Scott states he has had high blood pressure (HBP) for 15 years but that he has no other medical problems. He states he was taking 50 mg hydrochlorothiazide (HCTZ) and 50 mg Tenormin, each twice a day. Mr. Scott admits that 1 month ago he had stopped taking his medication for weeks while he had a cold, but he has been back on his medicine since. Mr. Scott states he last saw his doctor 10 months ago at which time his BP was above normal. At his last visit his doctor had said if the BP remained high, he would change Mr. Scott's medication at the next visit. Mr. Scott did not keep his follow-up appointment and states, "I do not like to go to the doctor." At triage Mr. Scott denies any headache, chest pain, shortness of breath, peripheral edema, extremity weakness, paresthesia, or visual changes.

Triage Assessment, Acuity Level II: high blood pressure, in no acute distress, BP systolic < 200, diastolic < 115; laceration with distal circulation, motor ability, and sensation (CMS) intact, hemostasis achieved by direct pressure.

In the treatment area Mr. Scott's repeat BP sitting is right arm 186/124, left arm 182/120, with a regular pulse of 76 beats/min. Mr. Scott's previous medical record reveals four ED visits over the past 2 years, all for miscellaneous chief complaints not related to high BP. During each visit his BP was elevated and he had been advised to continue his medications and keep his follow-up appointment to maintain BP control. Mr. Scott's funduscopic exam reveals arterial-venous (A-V) nicking bilaterally with sharp discs. His heart sounds are normal S1, S2; no S3, S4, or murmur; point of maximal impulse (PMI) is nondisplaced. His lungs are clear, his peripheral pulses are 4+, and there are no carotid, femoral, or renal bruits. There is no evidence of peripheral or sacral edema. A 12-lead ECG shows normal sinus rhythm without signs of myocardial ischemia or hypertrophy. A urinalysis shows 1+ protein and a specific gravity of 1.021. Chest x-ray reveals mild left ventricular hypertrophy. The electrolytes and CBC are normal.

Mr. Scott discussed his efforts at BP control over the years. He has decreased his cigarette smoking from three packs a day to three cigarettes a day. He denies the use of alcohol or illegal drugs. He says he eats in fast-food restaurants every day, though he understands that salt could increase his BP.

Mr. Scott was given 10 mg nifedipine sublingual. Within 30 min his BP decreased to 152/98 and was maintained at the lower level for over 1 hour. He was instructed at discharge to continue his 50 mg HCTZ twice a day, to discontinue the Tenormin, and begin enalapril 5 mg, 1/2 tablet each morning. Follow-up care was established using the departmental guidelines (Table 10.1). Mr. Scott was instructed to call his doctor and make an appointment to be seen within a week.

QUESTIONS AND ANSWERS

1. **Is there a relationship between Mr. Scott's elevated BP and possible anxiety induced by finger trauma?**

   Stressors such as a visit to the ED or finger trauma can cause increased sympathetic nervous system activity. Such activity may result in labile BP changes in which there is a diastolic BP greater than 90 mm Hg in an individual who usually has a diastolic BP less than 90 mm Hg (1). Mr. Scott, who has a documented 15-year history of HBP is not having labile BP changes. Of those patients with labile BP, it is estimated that 10 to 25% will progress to conditions of chronic HBP (1).

2. **What is the pathophysiological rationale for achieving and maintaining a normal BP in an otherwise asymptomatic patient?**

   There are two pathophysiological processes which occur during the asymptomatic or silent years of HBP. Trauma to the vessels in the arterial circulation occurs, causing accelerated atherosclerosis in large vessels and thinning and possible rupture of small vessels (1). In addition, HBP causes increased peripheral vascular resistance and increased work load on the heart (2). Patients can remain asymptomatic for years while target organ damage is occurring, primarily in the heart, kidneys, and cerebellum. Left ventricular hypertrophy can develop from cardiac adaptation to the increased pressure and afterload caused by the elevated BP (3,4). This was evident on Mr. Scott's chest x-ray. Enlargement of the left ventricle can produce myocardial ischemia, angina pectoris, congestive heart failure, and myocardial infarction. Arteriosclerosis of renal vessels can occur causing renal insufficiency and ultimately renal failure. Mr. Scott could be showing early renal disease, evidenced by the 1+ protein found on urinalysis. His long-standing HBP has caused the small vessels of the kidney, particularly the basement membrane of the glomerulus, to become thick and fibrotic, preventing effective filtration of metabolic wastes, resulting in proteinuria (3).

   Plaques and emboli can lead to hypertensive encephalopathy, cerebral hemorrhage, and stroke (2,5). The vascular changes from HBP within the eye result in retinopathy. As the pressure rises, the arterioles in the retina constrict and leak. Leaking can cause the formation of cotton wool spots, hemorrhages, and papilledema (3). Mr. Scott's funduscopic exam revealed early retinal changes associated with a history of long-standing elevated BP.

3. **Mr. Scott seems to understand some aspects of his disease, particularly by his effort to decrease his tobacco use. He continues, however, to**

avoid regular visits to his primary care provider, because he feels fine. What factors influence Mr. Scott's noncompliant behavior?

The dilemma of treatment compliance in HBP is that the majority of people who have the disease are symptom-free. It is estimated that 50% of patients with HBP drop out of their treatment program within the first year, and 75% within 5 years (6). Numerous socioeconomic factors can determine a person's ability to follow an HBP treatment program such as income, education, occupation, and race (7). Complexity of regimen has also been identified as a cofactor for noncompliance. Single-dose therapy has been found to have a greater influence on drug adherence than multiple dose therapies (8,9).

However, even before therapy can be established, the patient needs to have access into care, and once referred, appointment-keeping compliance. A needs assessment of both the patient and the system can identify factors that either enhance or impede a particular patient's compliance with treatment (10). The individual patient's coping skills and attitude toward himself and HBP have an obvious impact on subsequent behavior. The patient's social support system of family or friends is of value as is his ability to pay for care and medication (11). Lack of transportation to and from appointments may also influence appointment-keeping behavior. Preappointment reminders, in the form of phone calls or mailings, have been shown to enhance appointment-keeping behavior significantly (11,12,13). The greatest impact on patient compliance has been identified as the provider-patient relationship (14,15,16). Factors that have a positive influence on this relationship are that the patient see the same provider each visit, and that the provider convey a sense of having time for the patient, including the family, when possible. Discussion and instructions should be presented in language the patient can understand with opportunity for questions. In addition, the patient needs to know what the treatment program is as well as its purpose (17). Direct verbal communication of the information by the provider can usually produce greater compliance than written material (10). Mr. Scott displays some knowledge of HBP and the cardiovascular risk factors (i.e., smoking) but has not been compliant with follow-up care resulting in poorly controlled BP and early signs of target-organ damage.

4. **How does Mr. Scott's noncompliant behavior affect his mortality and morbidity from HBP?**

Mr. Scott is a middle-aged black male with a 15-year history of HBP, poorly controlled for at least 5 years, and showing evidence of early target-organ damage. In the United States HBP is more prevalent among blacks compared with whites and starts at an earlier age and has a higher incidence and mortality rate in blacks (3,18). In fact, the highest incidence of HBP is among middle-aged black males. The disease is more severe in blacks and causes more end-organ damage. This leads to a higher case fatality rate. Though mortality from HBP has been declining since 1950, it continues to show higher prevalence in the middle-aged black male population.

5. **What nursing diagnoses apply to this patient situation?**

Mr. Scott, though asymptomatic, has a sustained diastolic BP of around 115. He requires prompt evaluation and care. His management will focus on pharmacological intervention to decrease the BP without cardiovascular compromise. However, the greatest challenge lies in the education of the patient about this disease with appropriate referral for continuing care. The appropriate nursing diagnoses for this patient's care are (19):

Diagnosis: Potential for alteration in cardiac output related to increased systemic vascular resistance from vasoconstriction

Desired patient outcome: The patient's diastolic BP will be less than or equal to 80 to 100 mm Hg.

Diagnosis: Knowledge deficit related to HBP treatment and its asymptomatic target-organ damage.

Desired patient outcome: The patient will describe the relationship between elevated BP and damage to other body systems and will be symptom-free.

Diagnosis: Knowledge deficit related to HBP and its implications for life-style change.

Desired patient outcome: The patient will describe the relationship between his uncontrolled BP and poor compliance with medication and follow-up care, smoking, and dietary habits. The patient will stop smoking and describe measures to reduce salt intake.

Diagnosis: Noncompliance related to lack of understanding of benefits of maintaining treatment program.

Desired patient outcome: The patient will identify reason(s) for noncompliant behavior; the patient will acknowledge consequences of continued noncompliant behavior; the patient will participate in agreed-on plan of care.

6. **What nursing interventions should the nurse initiate in this situation?**

Nursing interventions for Mr. Scott have both a clinical and educational focus. The clinical goal is an acute and efficacious reduction in BP. The nurse should repeat the triage BP in both arms, establishing a baseline. Pertinent questions should be asked targeted at acute symptomatology related to increased BP such as chest pain, shortness of breath, peripheral edema, visual changes, and paresthesias. The nurse should perform a physical exam related to target-organ systems including the heart, lungs, and peripheral extremities. The physician will order a baseline ECG to evaluate the patient for ischemia and left ventricular hypertrophy that would influence choice of pharmacological intervention. The doctor ordered 10 mg nifedipine sublingual because of Mr. Scott's target-organ damage and elevated repeat BP. Nifedipine is a calcium-channel-blocking agent that produces prompt reduction of both systolic and diastolic BP, mean arterial pressure, and systemic vascular resistance (20,21). Onset of action of sublingual nifedipine is 55 to 10 min after administration. Maximal effect is achieved within 30 min, with a mean duration of action of 4 to 6 hr (20).

TIP: A reflex increase in heart rate occurs in most patients receiving sublingual nifedipine. Therefore, the nurse must closely monitor Mr. Scott's BP and pulse particularly for the first 15 min, and thereafter every half hour.

Possible adverse effects in the use of nifedipine include dizziness, headache, palpitation, premature ventricular beats, and hypotension (20). Mr. Scott's BP following treatment with nifedipine was 152/98, and he experienced no adverse effects. His stay in the ED was extended an additional hour to monitor his vital signs for any prolonged adverse effects of nifedipine.

The second area of importance for nursing intervention involves patient education. While Mr. Scott is having his vital signs monitored, the nurse can enhance a positive patient-provider relationship. This relationship is vital to Mr. Scott's compliance outcome (22). The nurse should close the door if possible, creating a few quiet moments to discuss BP in clear language appropriate for Mr. Scott. The nurse should recognize that the most vital area of noncompliance for Mr. Scott is his follow-up with a primary provider. The nurse should explore some of the factors specific to Mr. Scott's reasons for noncompliance and identify potential areas for assistance and improvement. Potential barriers to compliance such as cost, transportation, and scheduling conflicts with work or other responsibilities should be explored. The nurse should discuss reasons why Mr. Scott stopped taking his BP medication. The nurse should also review Mr. Scott's understanding of the role sodium intake plays in BP control. The nurse should review what foods Mr. Scott eats followed by what foods should be avoided. Since processed foods are consumed daily by Mr. Scott and are very high in sodium, they are of particular concern. Recipes that make food without salt appealing would be valuable. A referral to the dietician may be indicated.

Mr. Scott will need follow-up within a few weeks of discharge from the ED following pharmacological intervention. The nurse should refer Mr. Scott back to his usual source of care. Table 10.1.1 provides a guideline on HBP referral.

Table 10.1.1 High Blood Pressure Referral Guidelines[a]

Diastolic Blood Pressure	Follow-up within:	Systolic Blood Pressure When DBP < 90	Follow-up within:
		History of HBP	
< 90	2 months	< 140	2 months
90–104	2 months	140–199	2 months
≥ 105	1 week	≥ 200	1 week
≥ 115	48 hr		
		No History of HBP	
< 90	1 year	< 140	1 year
90 to 104	2 months	140–199	2 months
≥ 105	1 week	≥ 200	1 week
≥ 115	48 hr		

[a]Any HBP medication prescribed, modified, or given during ED visit, follow-up as per physician instructions (but not longer than 1 week).
Adapted from Report of the Joint National Committee on Detection, Evaluation, and Treatment of High Blood Pressure; approved by The East Baltimore High Blood Pressure Control Program and The Johns Hopkins Hospital Department of Emergency Medicine, with permission. Baltimore, The Johns Hopkins Hospital, 1988.

The nurse will provide Mr. Scott with needed information about the medications that were prescribed by the physician as well as about side effects. The nurse will describe the appropriate actions to take if unusual changes occur, such as chest pain or paresthesia. With the appropriate nurse-patient relationship the nurse should try to influence Mr. Scott to maintain his relationship with his primary doctor. All these aspects of patient education along with Mr. Scott's desire to change poor health behaviors will ultimately reduce his potential for mortality and morbidity.

REFERENCES

1. Barker L, Burton J, Zieve P: Principles of ambulatory medicine. 2nd ed. Baltimore: Williams & Wilkins, 1986.
2. Wyngarden J, Smith L: Cecil textbook of medicine. 17th ed. Philadelphia: Saunders, 1985.
3. Jackle M, Rasmussen C: Renal problems: A critical care nursing focus. London: Prentice-Hall, 1980.
4. Curry CL, Lewis JF: Cardiac anatomy and function in hypertensive blacks. In: Hall W, Saunders E, Shulman N, eds. Hypertension in blacks: Epidemiology, pathophysiology and treatment. Chicago: Year Book, 1985:61.
5. Snyder M, Jackle M: Neurologic problems: a critical care nursing focus. London: Prentice-Hall, 1981.
6. Cooper ES: Cerebrovascular disease in blacks. In: Hall W, Saunders E, Shulman N, eds. Hypertension in blacks: epidemiology, pathophysiology and treatment. Chicago: Year Book 1985:83.
7. Roter DL: Patient participation in the patient-provider interaction. *Health Educ Monogr* 1977;5(4):281.
8. Korsch B, Gozzi E, Francis V: Gaps in doctor-patient communication. *Pediatrics* 1968;42(5):855.
9. Prineas R, Gillum R: U.S. epidemiol-

ogy of hypertension in blacks. In: Hall W, Saunders E, Schulman N, eds. Hypertension in blacks: epidemiology, pathophysiology and treatment, Chicago: Year Book, 1985:17.

10. Anderson RJ, Kirk LM: Method of improving patient compliance in chronic disease states. *Arch Intern Med* 1982; 142:1673.

11. Haynes RB: Strategies to improve compliance with referrals, appointments, and prescribed medical regimens. In Haynes RB, Taylor DW, Sackett DL, eds. Compliance in health care. Baltimore: Johns Hopkins, 1979;121.

12. Bone L, Mamon J, Levine D, et al.: Emergency department detection and follow-up of high blood pressure: use and effectiveness of community health workers. *Am J Emerg Med* 1989;7:16.

13. Bone L, Levine D, Perry R, Marisky D, Green L: Update on the factors associated with high blood pressure compliance. *Md St Med J* 1984;33(3):201.

14. National High Blood Pressure Education Program. The 1988 report of the joint national committee on detection, evaluation and treatment of high blood pressure. (NIH Publication No. 88-1088). Washington, D.C.: National Institutes of Health, 1988.

15. Eastaugh SR, Hutcher ME: Improving compliance among hypertensives: A triage criterion with cost-benefit implications. *Med Care* 1982;20(10):1001.

16. Wagner E, Truesdale R, Warner J: Compliance, treatment practices and blood pressure control: community survey findings. *J Chronic Dis* 1981;34:519.

17. Gunter-Hunt G, Ferguson K, Bole G: Appointment-keeping behavior and patient satisfaction: implications for health professionals. *Patient Counsel Health Educ* 1979;3(4):156.

18. Blackwell B: The drug regimen and treatment compliance. In: Haynes RB, Taylor DW, Sackett DL, eds. Compliance in health care. Baltimore: Johns Hopkins, 1979:144.

19. Carpenito LJ: Nursing diagnosis, application to clinical practice. 2nd ed. New York: Lippincott, 1987.

20. Houston MC: The comparative effects of clonidine hydrochloride and nifedipine in the treatment of hypertensive crisis. *Am Heart J* 1988;115(1):152.

21. Hill MN, Cunningham SL: The latest words for high BP. *Am J Nurs* 1984; 89(4):504.

22. McCombs J, Fink J, Bandy P: Critical patient behaviors in a high blood pressure control. *Cardiovasc Nurs* 1980; 6(4):1–4.

10.2 CHEMICAL DEPENDENCE: MOVING TOWARD DETOX

Ronald Nichols, RN

Tom is a 37-year-old, divorced, white male who is brought to the ED by a concerned friend. Tom's friend states that Tom has been drinking heavily for weeks and has started to act strangely. He has locked himself in his apartment and has not gone outside for days. When the nurse speaks to Tom, he is alert and oriented to person and place. He does not know the day or date. Tom smells of ethanol (ETOH) and his affect is mildly restricted. His behavior in general is appropriate for an individual mildly intoxicated. Tom's triage vital signs are BP 134/84, pulse 88 and regular, respirations 18 and regular, temperature 98° F. Tom's pupils are equal and reactive to light. He has positive bilateral nystagmus. His physical exam is otherwise negative.

Tom denies any history of medical problems, takes no medications, and has no drug allergies. Tom states he has never before been treated for chemical dependency. He acknowledges that he has used cocaine intranasally on weekends since age 32.

He initially was using $80 a weekend and now is up to $240 "or so" for the last 6 months. He states he steals and sells drugs to support his habit. Tom states that he has thought about "mainlining" recently as he continues to crave cocaine more and feels "depressed" the day after using it. Drinking helps him feel better. Tom's usual ETOH intake is 2 six-packs of beer and a pint of whiskey daily. Tom states he has been drinking since he was 13 years old, became a weekend binger at age 18, and a daily drinker after his marriage failed. He has been drinking at his current rate for 1½ years.

Tom acknowledges that his father was an alcoholic and physically abused Tom as a child. Tom states he is "not like" his father and does not have a problem. Tom says he has stopped drinking on his own many times in the past. He just "likes to drink." Tom is able to share that, on occasion, when he stops drinking, he feels "ill," with shaking, sweating, nervousness, anorexia, nausea, vomiting, sleeping difficulties, and feeling paranoid. He denies seizures or hallucinations. He always feels much better "within a day or two" when he resumes drinking.

Tom's pattern of drinking includes a beer for breakfast, one or two beers for lunch "just to get by" and "no real heavy" drinking until he gets home from work. Tom admits that he was fired from his job 2 weeks ago and is about to be evicted from his apartment. He states his family "hates" him and will not speak to him when he calls. He has been arrested once for driving while intoxicated (DWI). Tom admits that he has recently thought of killing himself but has made no specific plans or attempts. Tom states he drank a pint of whiskey and "snorted coke" late last night. He only came to the ED today because his friend asked him to.

Triage Assessment, Acuity Level III: alcohol and drug dependence; potential for acute withdrawal.

Tom is taken to the treatment area to begin medical management for alcohol and cocaine withdrawal and to initiate a referral for detoxification.

QUESTIONS AND ANSWERS

1. **What is the first priority in nursing and medical management of the substance-abuse patient?**

   Patients who abuse alcohol and other drugs need to be assessed for their degree of dependence and the physical compromises that may have occurred with chronic abuse. Tom relates a typical case history of chronic abuse for many years. He clearly has had problems with serious withdrawal symptoms when he has attempted to stop drinking in the past.

   The focus of nursing and medical therapy should be to help Tom through the initial withdrawal phase of chemical dependency with particular attention to preventing injury. Acute alcohol withdrawal can lead to death. Lab tests will usually indicate serious chemical imbalances including glucose, magnesium, calcium, and liver enzymes. Tom should initially be treated with fluids, magnesium sulfate, Folvite, and other electrolytes as needed. He should also be provided with PO sedation to aid in the control of tremors, nervousness, and hallucinations, all hallmarks of acute withdrawal syndrome.

The benzodiazepines seem to be the safest and most effective chemical agents for reducing alcohol withdrawal symptoms.

Tom has expressed some concern about feelings of suicide, which is not unusual during acute alcohol intoxication. Therefore, he should be managed in a highly visible, well-lighted area. Restraint as an initial intervention is discouraged but may become necessary, if in the course of withdrawal, Tom threatens harm to himself or others.

TIP: In some instances patients do not require direct medical management for acute detoxification. If the home situation is supportive, a family member can help the patient with medications, fluids, and diet. A social worker may be needed to help assess the home environment or to help place the patient in an appropriate shelter.

As Tom completes this initial phase of withdrawal, which may last for several hours, a complete medical exam is indicated. Particular attention should be paid to the neurological exam to rule out head trauma or other pathologies that may be contributing to Tom's altered mental state and psychiatric symptoms.

2. **Once Tom has been helped through the acute withdrawal phase from alcohol and cocaine, what then? Alcoholics and drug addicts just come back and clog up our ED. What can we do?**

A caring, nonjudgmental, nonconfronting attitude by the nurse while carrying out nursing activities is the first step to establishing a trusting, therapeutic relationship. Patients with problems related to substance abuse are used to being told they are "hopeless," "have no motivation," "going to die." They are used to being mistreated. The substance abuser usually has a "crisis" orientation to life situations and is seen in the ED secondary to some other real or perceived crisis, not usually for their substance-abuse problem. Even if the person is able to ask for help for their abuse problem, they are not always able to move beyond recognition of need.

Chemical dependency is a disease and must be approached as such by everyone involved in the patient's care. Chemical dependence should not be approached as a "moral weakness," "lack of will power," or even "desired" life-style. The substance abuser did not take his first drink or injection with the intent of addiction. Addiction results from a combination of genetics and environment. Cocaine, nicotine, and heroin seem to be the most addictive drugs used today, with relapse rates approaching 100%. Most often, relapse can be traced to the environment and cues which set off internal stimuli for drug craving, such as pictures, talk of "using" or drinking, and physical and psychological distress.

For many people substance abuse has become such a way of life that they do not know how to quit. Most substance-abuse patients have not been drug-free since adolescence. Many substance-abuse patients cannot say why they started, why they have problems with relapse, or why they want to quit. Motivation for treatment is very hard to establish and is frequently associated with the most recent crisis that brought the individual to the ED. Even if motivation is established, success is not guaranteed. Relapse should be considered a normal, expected part of the disease, much like hypoglycemia is a common recurrence with a patient with diabetes mellitus.

3. **Denial is a big obstacle to patient development of motivation. How can an ED nurse with episodic contact with the patient help him to recognize there is a problem?**

Denial is a natural part of being human: the patient with chest pain who refuses to be evaluated, the hypertensive patient with headaches who does not take his medication, the young executive with a family history of colorectal cancer who cannot find time for an annual physical. All these people believe that "I" am not sick; it is always "the other" person.

In many instances, the substance abuser in the ED cannot remember why he came to the ED (blackouts) or may have cognitive or learning disabilities that are genetic or the result of many years of substance abuse. The patient's ability to acknowledge that there is a problem is very limited under these circumstances. In many instances, acknowledgment of a problem occurs only gradually.

The ability to rationally accept that there is a problem and effectively do something about it may take even longer. This slow realization process is one reason why there is a high level of recidivism from 5- to 7-day treatment programs. However, each time the patient returns for help there may be a new level of appreciation by the patient for his problem that may enhance his motivation for the next time.

4. **What are the appropriate nursing diagnoses for this patient?**

Besides the nursing problems related to his physiological needs, the patient with a substance-abuse problem has many psychosocial needs. These are usually specific to the patient and his constellation of support persons. For Tom who has not had family support for some time, the nursing diagnoses may be made as follows:

Diagnose: Self-esteem disturbance related to history of poor out-

comes in social interactions evidenced by suicidal feelings; lack of social supports.

<u>Desired patient outcome:</u> The patient will identify internal and external stimuli that contribute to feelings of unworthiness; the patient will identify internal and external resources that will assist him to develop more positive feelings about himself; the patient will describe the role alcohol and cocaine play in enhancing feelings of depression and poor self-esteem.

Diagnosis: Potential for self-directed violence related to stated feelings of depression enhanced by chronic substance abuse

<u>Desired patient outcome:</u> The patient will describe improved mood, increased hopefulness, and decreased suicidal ideation or intent; the patient will identify internal or external resources that he can use when these feelings occur; the patient will describe the role alcohol and cocaine play in enhancing these feelings.

Diagnosis: Ineffective individual coping related to inability to make appropriate decisions in health care enhanced by chronic substance abuse

<u>Desired patient outcome:</u> The patient will identify internal and environmental stressors which impair his ability to make appropriate health care decisions; the patient will verbalize an understanding of how alcohol and cocaine interfere with his ability to make appropriate decisions; the patient will identify personal strengths that may promote effective coping and decision making in a situational crisis.

Diagnosis: Social isolation related to self-imposed withdrawal enhanced by chronic alcohol and drug use

<u>Desired patient outcome:</u> The patient will not isolate himself from friends and relatives; the patient will state why social interaction is necessary; the patient will identify one person he will call when he feels the need to lock himself in his apartment.

The nurse working with the substance-abuse patient in the acute-care setting should work with the counselors and other health care providers to help the patient accept treatment, regardless of his willingness to agree that there is a problem. The patient should be told that he is not responsible for his disease but that he is responsible for his recovery. The nurse should support his family and friends to take on a "tough love" attitude toward the patient. The feeling conveyed should be that "I will help you to work on solutions to the problem; I will not help you to find excuses or help you to die." The nurse in the ED should not fight the patient's denial. The nurse should provide nonreactive emotional support to the patient and make the patient aware of available treatment. The patient will decide when he is ready to help himself.

SUGGESTED READINGS

Aderhold RN, Mooring RA: Alcoholism. In: Dornbrand L, Hooli AJ, Fletcher RH, and Picard Jr GG, eds. Manual of clinical problems in adult ambulatory care. Boston: Little, Brown, 1985:456.

Clark WD: Alcoholism: Blocks to diagnosis and treatment. *Am J Med* 1981;71: 275–286.

Finley B: Counseling the alcoholic client. *J Psychiat Nurs* 1981;19:32–34.

Svitlik B: Helping the alcoholic patient on the road to recovery. *J Emerg Nurs* 1980; 7(8):119–203.

10.3 WHEN THE DIAGNOSIS IS AIDS

Karla Alwood, MS, CRNP

Joann is a 27-year-old black female who presents to the triage nurse of the Emergency Department complaining of a sore throat progressively worsening over the past 2 weeks. She reports that the throat pain is now so severe that she is unable to eat solid food and is even having difficulty swallowing fluids. Joann describes some mild upper respiratory symptoms that include congestion, rhinitis, and a loose, mildly productive cough of clear to white sputum. She has also noted slight dyspnea on exertion. She denies any nausea, vomiting, or diarrhea but complains of occasional chills and sweats at night. In addition, Joann describes a history of fatigue that has persisted and gradually worsened over the past 3 to 4 months.

Joann's report of her past medical history is vague. She denies any major medical problems or hospitalizations. She states that she was treated for a rash on her back approximately 1 year ago and has a history of a "low blood count." She admits to previous intravenous drug use and sharing needles but states she has been relatively drug free for the past month. She occasionally drinks alcohol but denies recent ingestion because it burns her throat. She has no regular medical provider and seeks episodic health care through the emergency department.

On brief examination, the triage nurse notes a thin black female, mildly ill appearing. Her BP is 94/60, HR 110, temperature 100.6°F. Her respirations are 20 and easy. She has tender, enlarged cervical lymph nodes bilaterally. Her tonsils are not swollen, but the pharynx is red and covered with a white exudate. There is no trismus and, despite her pain with swallowing, she has no difficulty handling her secretions. She has scarred tract marks on both arms and mildly dry scaling areas on her face and hairline.

Triage Assessment, Acuity Level I: Sore throat, upper respiratory infection (URI) symptoms, RR < 32, fever < 102.

The patient is referred to the "non-urgent" clinic for further care. There, a more detailed history is taken. Joann describes a burning sensation with swallowing that travels all the way down to her stomach. The night sweats she had related earlier have been occurring off and on for over a year, but have recently worsened with the onset of her current symptoms. She has not taken her temperature but reports that the sweats have been occurring 4 to 5 nights of the week to the extent that she has to get up and change her night clothes and bed linen. Her dyspnea has also been gradually worsening over the past few months, and some days she feels too tired even to get out of bed. Her URI symptoms started about 2 months ago but have not worsened, and her cough, although mildly productive, remains clear. Of additional concern to her is a progressive, unexplained weight loss that started about 6 months ago and now totals approximately 20 lb.

Joann states that her dry, scaling skin rashes have persisted despite the use of emollients. She states that she has been taking over-the-counter (OTC) iron pills for her low blood count. Her last menstrural period was approximately 1 month ago and she notes occasional menstrural irregularities that are not new. She denies a history of sexually transmitted diseases but reports frequent vaginal yeast infections over the past year. She has a steady sexual partner who also uses intravenous drugs, and she uses no regular form of contraception. She denies drug allergies or use of prescription medications. She smokes 1 pack of cigarettes per day and drinks alcohol occasionally. She has a 5-year history of intravenous drug use (IVDU) and last used intravenous drugs approximately 2 to 3 weeks ago. She shares needles only with her sex partner. An old chart reveals that the rash she described a year ago was diagnosed as shingles (herpes zoster). At that time, due to her presenting history and diagnoses, she was counseled and tested for human immunodeficiency virus (HIV). She failed to keep her follow-up appointment despite numerous attempts made to contact her. Joann is currently unaware that her enzyme-linked immunosorbent assay (ELISA) and Western blot tests were positive.

QUESTIONS AND ANSWERS

1. **What is the etiology of the past and present medical history of this patient?**

    When Joann presented with herpes zoster a year ago she was experiencing symptoms of immune suppression. Depressed cellular immunity in conjunction with her history of intravenous drug use and sharing of needles is a predictor for HIV and acquired immune deficiency syndrome (AIDS) (1).

    The etiologic agent of AIDS is HIV. This virus induces a progressive, time-dependent destruction of T4 lymphocytes, which are key components to the integrity of the cellular immune system (2). In addition, the virus has been found to invade other classes of immune cells such as cells of the nervous system, intestine, kidney, and bone marrow. This, in part, accounts for the widespread and complex nature of an HIV infection. With progressive viral invasion and destruction of lymphocytes, cellular immunity declines, and the opportunistic infections that characterize this disease begin to emerge.

    The HIV-infected patient often presents with symptoms that indicate a predictable, progressive derangement of immune function, with AIDS being a late manifestation of that process. The specific stages of HIV infection may be viewed on a continuum that chart the decline of the immune system. Initially, the majority of individuals infected with HIV are asymptomatic, although some may experience a mononucleosis-like illness that will completely resolve, persist, or evolve into one of the other HIV-associated syndromes. Throughout the course of HIV infection, various constitutional symptoms or the so-called AIDS related complex (ARC) may develop. These symptoms are characterized by persistent generalized lymphadenopathy, unexplained fevers, persistent night sweats, chronic diarrhea, and weight loss. Additional manifestations with a somewhat poorer prognosis include oral candidiasis, hairy leukoplakia, immune thrombocytopenia, and multidermatomal herpes zoster (3).

This disease has a long latency or subclinical phase that, according to recent reports, may persist up to 10 years (3). However, as T4 cell counts decline, infected persons exhibit increasingly more overt symptomatology indicative of immune dysfunction. End-stage disease or AIDS is usually seen when the T4 cell count falls below 200 (400 to 1600 is normal) and opportunistic infections emerge. Some of the more common or virulent forms of infection found in the United States include *Pneumocystis carinii* pneumonia, parasitic infections such as toxoplasmosis and cryptosporidiosis, fungal infections such as cryptococcosis and histoplasmosis, and viruses such as cytomegalovirus and chronic mucocutaneous herpes simplex. Other AIDS-defining illnesses include Kaposi's sarcoma, some forms of lymphoma, wasting syndrome, and AIDS encephalopathy (3).

2. **What are the ELISA and Western blot blood tests and what do they diagnose?**

The ELISA test identifies HIV antibodies. In the asymptomatic patient, a positive ELISA test is an indication of exposure and infection with HIV, but is not diagnostic for AIDS. The Western blot analysis uses electrophoretically marked proteins to differentiate antibodies and is used in conjunction with the ELISA test to confirm a diagnosis of HIV. AIDS is defined when an opportunistic infection or cancer presents in the HIV-infected individual.

TIP: A patient with a positive HIV test does not necessary have AIDS. This distinction is important when providing counseling and making patient referrals. However, it is important to note that patients may be severely immunocompromised and still remain asymptomatic, emphasizing the need for prompt medical follow-up.

---

3. **What are the risk factors for HIV acquisition and transmission in this patient? How can future HIV transmission be avoided?**

Transmission of HIV occurs primarily through three known routes: (*a*) inoculation of blood by transfusion of blood or blood products, needle sharing among intravenous drug users, and needle stick, open wound, and mucous membrane exposure in health care workers; (*b*) sexual activity with known HIV-infected or high-risk partners; and (*c*) perinatal, intrauterine, or peripartum exposure (4). Joann has two of these risk factors (sexual partner and IVDU) and poses a potential threat to future offspring since she is not currently using any regular form of contraception.

Transmission of the HIV virus may be easily prevented in all three of these situations. First, needle sharing among intravenous drug users should be avoided in all instances. If this is not possible, all needle works should be cleaned in bleach prior to each use. Safer sex practices using latex condoms with nonoxynol 9 spermicidal foam or jelly should prevent both pregnancy and sexual transmission of disease. In addition, condoms and foam prevent transmission of other sexually transmitted diseases (5, 6).

4. **What nursing diagnoses are most applicable to this situation?**

Nursing diagnoses for Joann are multiple and complex. First there are the problems related to her current physical needs. In addition, the actual and potential problems related to her HIV status combined with the psychological impact of receiving this information will require immediate and supportive attention. Although many of these problems cannot be solved during this visit, the nurse should enumerate primary concerns on the care plan and begin to systematically approach those that are of highest priority during this visit.

Diagnosis: Fluid volume deficit related to decreased fluid intake because of dysphagia, odynophagia, and repeated episodes of night sweats and fever.

Desired patient outcome: The patient will have improved skin turgor, moist mucous membranes, alert mental status, and BP systolic > 90 mm Hg and HR < 100.

Diagnosis: Altered nutrition, less than body requirements, related to the constitutional symptoms of HIV infection including anorexia, diarrhea, and decreased nutrient absorption.

Desired patient outcome: The patient will maintain her weight and develop strategies aimed at increasing her calorie intake. The patient will state ways to prepare high-calorie, high-protein foods or use supplements; prepare food so that it is visually appealing and provide herself with small, frequent, nutritional meals.

Diagnosis: Impaired swallowing related to irritation, pain, and swelling of esophagus and pharynx from presumed esophageal infection.

Desired patient outcome: The patient will have reduction in pain and improved ability to swallow. The patient will describe strategies for preparing very cold or warm fluids that will be more comfortable to swallow.

Diagnosis: *Activity intolerance related to anemia and imbalance between oxygen supply and demand from opportunistic infection.*

Desired patient outcome: The patient will describe strategies for conserving energy and provide the time and setting for adequate rest and sleep periods.

Diagnosis: *Knowledge deficit related to HIV and AIDS and implications for health, health management, and prognosis.*

Desired patient outcome: The patient will be able to describe what an HIV infection is, how to recognize worrisome signs and symptoms, and how to prevent transmission to others by using safe sex practices and by not sharing needles.

Diagnosis: *Potential for impaired adjustment related to required changes in life-style to maintain wellness.*

Desired patient outcome: The patient will acknowledge the importance of life-style changes; the patient will state ways to remove barriers that impede change; the patient will identify personal strengths that will aid her in making life-style changes; and the patient will follow-up on her care.

Diagnosis: *Potential for anticipatory grieving related to poor prognosis associated with AIDS.*

Desired patient outcome: The patient will be able to discuss her potential loss and will begin the experience of grieving in a supportive environment. The patient will verbalize that grief is "normal" secondary to loss. The patient will identify grieving behavior, such as variability in mood and preoccupation, as normal and will develop strategies to accept and modify these.

Diagnosis: *Potential for body image disturbance related to body changes that occur with AIDS complications such as continued weight loss, hair loss, development of skin lesions, and so on.*

Desired patient outcome: The patient will describe strategies to visually enhance body image through use of dress, hair covering, and covering of wounds. The patient will describe coping mechanisms and social supports for this process.

Diagnosis: *Potential for impaired social interaction related to behavior of social supports and others that may fear infection from social contact or criticize social behavior of intravenous drug use.*

Desired patient outcome: The patient will demonstrate behavior that may maintain or improve social interactions; the patient will practice "safe" behavior that will communicate to others that she is being responsible (i.e., safe sex, use of disposable tissues when coughing, no needle sharing, contraception, etc.).

Other diagnoses that may be considered are:

Anxiety
Potential for chronic pain
Sleep pattern disturbance
Potential for new infections
Altered wake-sleep patterns
Self-esteem disturbance

Potential family problems include:

Ineffective family coping: disabling or compromised
Potential for altered role performance

5. **What nursing interventions should the nurse initiate in this situation?**
In collaboration with the physician, the nurse should participate in the treatment of this patient's current infection. Antibiotic therapy should be initiated and an anti-inflammatory agent should be prescribed to reduce fever and provide comfort. The patient should be instructed on the use of these medications and the need for fluids. Given her current state of discomfort, dysphagia, and significant weight loss the nurse can recommend dietary strategies to improve her current nutritional deficits. A social worker should be consulted if the patient has significant social and financial constraints.

One of the more difficult aspects of Joann's care is providing support when she is informed of her HIV test results. Since Joann was tested a year ago, she must have considered the possibility of AIDS diagnosis. Her reasons for not following through are unknown; however, denial is often a normal reaction to a potentially unpleasant outcome. The supportive relationship that is established at the time she is told of her diagnosis should help her to move toward acknowledgment of her problem and the need for follow-up care. She should be encouraged that patients receiving appropriate medical care have a better long-term prognosis.

A "lifeline" should be provided to the patient including telephone numbers of HIV clinics and community agencies concerned with HIV patients. The reactions of family members and friends may be unpredictable, and the patient's permission to include them in the counseling and support role is required. For Joann, her boyfriend is an important link. He too may be infected and may require the same help and support as Joann. A patient such as Joann should be assisted to recognize and cope with the emotional feelings that accompany the diagnosis of AIDS. These feelings may include shock or disbelief; fear and anxiety related to prognosis and potential disability and abandonment; depression over the absence of a cure and inevitable physical decline; anger and concern over needed life-style changes; guilt related to possibly spreading the infection to others and acknowledgment of high-risk behavior such as intravenous drug use (7).

Joann needs regular follow-up care. Given her poor compliance in the past, the nurse should stress to Joann the need for regular medical follow-up. Many times, transportation and financial constraints are barriers to treatment that can be minimized through social work support. If at all possible the emergency department nurse can help the patient make the follow-up appointment with the AIDS counseling center. The nurse can help initiate a plan of care for the patient by providing the intake counselor at the follow-up center with the nursing diagnosis list already prepared and provide the counselor with a telephone number or significant other that can help to ensure follow-up compliance by the patient.

Joann should recover from her current illness and return to most of her normal activities. However, she must be committed to stopping her intravenous drug use and beginning a treatment program to maximize her long-term survival.

REFERENCES

1. Millize M, Goldert J, et al.: Risk of AIDS after herpes zoster. *Lancet* 1987;1:728–730.
2. Glatt AE, Chirgwin K, Landesman S: Treatment of infections associated with human immunodeficiency virus. *N Engl J Med* 1988;318:1439–1448.
3. Redfield R, Burke D: HIV infection. The science of AIDS: the clinical picture. In: Readings from Scientific American. New York: WH Freeman, 1988:63–75.
4. Revision of the CDC surveillance case definition for acquired immunodeficiency syndrome. *MMWR* 1987;36(15):3S–12S.
5. Friedland G, Klein R: Transmission of the human immunodeficiency virus. *N Engl J Med* 1987;317:1125–1133.
6. Hook EW: Syphilis and HIV infection. *J Infect Dis* 1989;160:530–534.
7. Miller D: ABC of AIDS: counseling. *Br Med J* 1987;294:1071–1074.

INDEX

Page numbers in *italics* denote figures; those followed by "t" denote tables.

239